50 LANDMARK PAPERS

every

Trauma Surgeon Should Know

50 LANDMARK PAPERS

every

Trauma Surgeon Should Know

EDITORS

Stephen M. Cohn, MD, FACS

Department of Surgery
Hackensack Meridian School of Medicine, Nutley, New Jersey

Ara J. Feinstein, MD, MPH, FACS

Associate Professor of Surgery
University of Arizona COM-PHX
Trauma, Emergency Surgery and Critical Care
Banner University Medical Center, Phoenix, Arizona

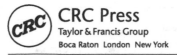

CRC Press
Taylor & Francis Group
Boca Raton London New York

CRC Press is an imprint of the
Taylor & Francis Group, an **informa** business

CRC Press
Taylor & Francis Group
6000 Broken Sound Parkway NW, Suite 300
Boca Raton, FL 33487-2742

© 2020 by Taylor & Francis Group, LLC
CRC Press is an imprint of Taylor & Francis Group, an Informa business

No claim to original U.S. Government works

Printed on acid-free paper

International Standard Book Number-13: 978-1-138-50674-9 (Hardback)
International Standard Book Number-13: 978-1-138-50629-9 (Paperback)

Library of Congress Cataloging-in-Publication Data

Names: Cohn, Stephen M., editor. | Feinstein, Ara J., editor.
Title: 50 landmark papers every trauma surgeon should know / [edited by]
Stephen M. Cohn and Ara J. Feinstein.
Other titles: Fifty landmark papers every trauma surgeon should know
Description: Boca Raton : CRC Press, [2018] | Includes bibliographical
references.
Identifiers: LCCN 2017060345 (print) | LCCN 2017058917 (ebook) | ISBN
9781138506299 (pbk. : alk. paper) | ISBN 9781138506749 (hardback : alk.
paper) | ISBN 9781315147017 (General eBook)
Subjects: | MESH: Wounds and Injuries--surgery | Surgical Procedures,
Operative--methods | Traumatology--methods | Review
Classification: LCC RD93 (ebook) | LCC RD93 (print) | NLM WO 700 | DDC
617.044--dc23
LC record available at https://lccn.loc.gov/2017060345

Visit the Taylor & Francis Web site at
http://www.taylorandfrancis.com

and the CRC Press Web site at
http://www.crcpress.com

Contents

Section One   Prehospital Trauma

Section Two   Trauma Bay

Section Three   Operating Room

Section Four   Hospital and Beyond

Preface

T he care of the patient who has suffered traumatic injury goes back as far as human history. And yet, the scientific underpinnings of our current management are far more recent. Trauma care has become a burgeoning field of scientific inquiry. Increasingly, the management of our patients is informed by evidence-based medicine and rigorous data analysis. But all this progress had to start somewhere. We chose these papers, albeit subjectively, because they underpin the daily care of our patients. Some of these practices are simply taken for granted, despite the ingenuity and audacity to make them a part of our armamentarium. There is no dearth of practitioners with big ideas, but few posses the fortitude to carry them through to a published manuscript. Over time, these articles changed the way we practice, and in doing so, continue to improve the lives of countless patients. In this volume, we attempt to both recognize and understand the process of innovation. We also seek to relate our history to our current practice. In doing so, we hope to inspire both a more evidence-based approach and provide a blueprint for reaching further. We endeavor to inspire and encourage surgeons to be receptive to change in the tireless effort to improve the care of our patients. The next revolutions in Trauma are waiting to be discovered and embraced.

Stephen M. Cohn
Ara J. Feinstein

Editors

Ara J. Feinstein is an Arizona native and graduated summa cum laude from the University of Arizona, Tucson. He received his MD from Yale University School of Medicine, New Haven, Connecticut, and trained in General Surgery at Massachusetts General Hospital. He completed an NIH-sponsored research fellowship and received a Masters in Public Health from the University of Miami, Coral Gables, Florida. His clinical fellowship in Trauma and Critical Care was at Ryder Trauma Center in Miami.

He is currently an Associate Professor of Surgery at the University of Arizona College of Medicine–Phoenix and serves as a Physician Executive, overseeing Specialty Care for Banner Medical Group.

Stephen M. Cohn began his academic career at University of Massachusetts Medical School after studying at Baylor College of Medicine, the University of California, and Boston University/Boston City Hospital. He joined Yale University School of Medicine as Chief of the Trauma Service until he was called to serve with the US Army Medical Corp in Desert Storm.

Upon return to New Haven, Dr. Cohn assumed the position as Division Chief of Trauma and Surgical Critical Care where he established a successful ACS level I trauma center, a surgical critical care fellowship, and an active research program. He subsequently moved to the University of Miami where he led the Divisions of Trauma and Surgical Critical Care as the Medical Director of the Ryder Trauma Center.

Dr. Cohn later served as Chairman of the Department of Surgery at the University of Texas Health Science Center at San Antonio. He now lives in New York City where he recently transitioned to the faculty of the new Hackensack/Meridian School of Medicine at Seton Hall as a clinician, educator, and researcher.

Contributors

Suresh "Mitu" Agarwal
Division of Trauma and Critical Care
  Surgery
Department of Surgery
Duke University School of Medicine
Durham, North Carolina

Hasan B. Alam
Department of Surgery
University of Michigan
Ann Arbor, Michigan

Susan P. Baker
Department of Surgery
The Johns Hopkins School of Public
  Health
Baltimore, Maryland

Philip S. Barie
Department of Surgery
Department of Public Health in Medicine
Weill Cornell Medicine
NewYork-Presbyterian Hospital/Weill
  Cornell Medical Center
New York, New York

Walter L. Biffl
Trauma and Acute Care Surgery
Scripps Memorial Hospital La Jolla
La Jolla, California

John Kennedy Bini
Department of Surgery
Boonshoft School of Medicine
Wright State University
and
Miami Valley Hospital
Dayton, Ohio
and
Department of Surgery
Uniformed Services University
Bethesda, Maryland

James N. Bogert
Division of Trauma
Department of Surgery
St. Joseph Hospital and Medical Center
Creighton University College
  of Medicine – Phoenix Campus
Phoenix, Arizona

Robert F. Buckman
Operative Experience, Inc.
North East, Maryland

Eileen M. Bulger
Department of Surgery
University of Washington
and
Harborview Medical Center
Seattle, Washington

Andrew R. Burgess
Department of Orthopaedic Surgery
McGovern Medical School at Houston
University of Texas
Houston, Texas

Peter A. Burke
Department of Surgery
Boston University School of Medicine
and
Boston Medical Center
Boston, Massachusetts

Howard R. Champion
Department of Surgery
Uniformed Services University of the
  Health Sciences
and
SimQuest
Bethesda, Maryland

Michael L. Cheatham
Orlando Health Physicians Surgical
  Group
Orlando Regional Medical Center
Orlando, Florida

Randall M. Chesnut
Department of Neurotrauma
and
Department of Neurological Surgery
and
Department of Orthopaedic Surgery
School of Global Health
University of Copenhagen
Copenhagen, Denmark

W. Darrin Clouse
Division of Vascular and Endovascular
  Surgery
Department of Surgery
Harvard Medical School
and
Massachusetts General Hospital
Boston, Massachusetts

Raul Coimbra
Department of Surgery
University of California San Diego
San Diego, California

Martin A. Croce
Regional One Health
Division of Trauma and Surgical
  Critical Care
Department of Surgery
University of Tennessee Health Science
  Center
Memphis, Tennessee

James W. Davis
Department of Clinical Surgery
University of California San Francisco
Medical Center
Fresno, California

E. Patchen Dellinger
Department of Surgery
University of Washington
Seattle, Washington

Demetrios Demetriades
Department of Surgery
University of Southern California
Los Angeles, California

Matthew O. Dolich
Department of Surgery
University of California Irvine Medical
  Center
Orange, California

Joseph J. DuBose
Baltimore Center for the Sustainment of
Trauma and Readiness Skills (CSTARS)
and
Uniformed Services University of the
  Health Sciences
and
University of Maryland School of
  Medicine
Baltimore, Maryland

Alexander L. Eastman
US Department of Homeland Security
Washington, DC

Brian J. Eastridge
Department of Surgery
Trauma and Emergency General Surgery
UT Health San Antonio
San Antonio, Texas

Timothy C. Fabian
Department of Surgery
University of Tennessee Health Sciences
  Center
Memphis, Tennessee

Samir M. Fakhry
Department of Surgery
George Washington University
Washington, DC
and
Trauma and Acute Care Surgery
Synergy Surgicalists
Reston Hospital Center
Reston, Virginia

Michael P. Federle
Department of Radiology
Stanford University School of Medicine
Stanford, California

David V. Feliciano
Department of Surgery
University of Maryland School
  of Medicine
and
Shock Trauma Center
Department of Surgery
University of Maryland Medical Center
Baltimore, Maryland

Paula Ferrada
Department of Surgery
Virginia Commonwealth University
Richmond, Virginia

Lewis Flint
Division of Education
American College of Surgeons
Chicago, Illinois

Kevin N. Foster
Department of Surgery
Maricopa Medical Center
Phoenix, Arizona

Asaf A. Gave
Department of Surgery
Hofstra School of Medicine
and
Staten Island University Hospital
Northwell Health
New York, New York

Larry M. Gentilello (Retired)

Alden H. Harken
East Bay Surgery Program
Department of Surgery
University of California San Francisco
San Francisco, California

Paul C. Hébert
Centre hospitalier de l'Université de
  Montréal
Department of Medicine (Critical Care)
University of Montréeal
and
CHUM Research Centre
Hema Quebec Bayer
University of Montréeal
Canadian Critical Care Trials Group
Montréal, Québec, Canada

David N. Herndon
Department of Surgery
University of Texas Medical Branch
Galveston, Texas

Kevin S. Hirsch
Department of Radiology
University of Arizona College of Medicine
Phoenix, Arizona

John B. Holcomb
Department of Surgery
Center for Translational Injury Research
McGovern Medical School
Houston, Texas

David B. Hoyt
Department of Surgery
American College of Surgeons
Chicago, Illinois

Parker J. Hu
Division of Acute Care Surgery
Department of Surgery
University of Alabama
Birmingham, Alabama

Rao R. Ivatury
Department of Surgery
Virginia Commonwealth University
Richmond, Virginia

Lenworth Jacobs
Department of Surgery
Trauma Institute
Hartford Hospital University of Connecticut
Mansfield, Connecticut

Donald H. Jenkins
Division of Trauma and Emergency
    Surgery
Military Health Institute
San Antonio, Texas

Kaj Johansen
Department of Surgery
University of Washington School of
    Medicine
Seattle, Washington

Clifford B. Jones
The CORE Institute
Orthopaedic Trauma and Bone Health
and
Department of Orthopaedic Surgery
University Arizona College of Medicine
and
Banner Health Orthopaedic Spine
    Institute
Trauma and Bone Health
Phoenix, Arizona

Bellal A. Joseph
Department of Surgery
University of Arizona
Tucson, Arizona

Gregory J. Jurkovich
Department of Surgery
University of California Davis
Sacramento, California

Riyad Karmy-Jones
Department of Trauma
Legacy Emanuel Medical Center Portland
Portland, Oregon
and
Thoracic and Vascular Surgery Peace
Health Southwest Washington Medical
    Center
Vancouver, Washington

Jeffrey D. Kerby
Division of Acute Care Surgery
Department of Surgery
University of Alabama
Birmingham, Alabama

Natasha Keric
University of Arizona College of
   Medicine–Phoenix Trauma
Banner–University Medical Center
Phoenix, Arizona

David R. King
Department of Surgery
Harvard Medical School
and
Division of Trauma, Emergency
   Surgery, and Surgical Critical Care
Massachusetts General Hospital
Boston, Massachusetts

Jeffrey H. Lawson
Department of Surgery
Duke University
and
Humacyte, Inc.
Durham, North Carolina

Frank R. Lewis
American Board of Surgery
Philadelphia, Pennsylvania

David H. Livingston
Division of Trauma and Surgical
   Critical Care
Department of Surgery
Rutgers New Jersey Medical School
Newark, New Jersey

Robert C. Mackersie
Trauma Center
University of California San Francisco
and
Department of Surgery
Zuckerberg San Francisco General
   Hospital
San Francisco, California

Mark A. Malangoni
General Surgeon
Bryn Mawr, Pennsylvania

Michael N. Margolies
Department of Surgery
Harvard Medical School
and
Massachusetts General Hospital
Boston, Massachusetts

John C. Marshall
Department of Surgery
University of Toronto
and
St. Michael's Hospital
Li Ka Shing Knowledge Institute
Ontario, Toronto, Canada

Kenneth L. Mattox
Department of Surgery
Baylor College of Medicine
Houston, Texas

Addison K. May
General Surgeon
Charlotte, North Carolina

J. Wayne Meredith
Department of Surgery
University of Louisville
Louisville, Kentucky

Anthony A. Meyer
Department of Surgery
University of North Carolina
Chapel Hill, North Carolina

Ernest E. Moore
Department of Surgery
Ernest E. Moore Shock Trauma Center
   at Denver Health
University of Colorado Denver
Denver, Colorado

Frederick A. Moore
Division of Acute Care Surgery
Department of Surgery
University of Florida
Gainesville, Florida

John A. Morris
Department of Surgery
Vanderbilt University Medical Center
Nashville, Tennessee

Felipe Múnera
Department of Radiology
Radiology Services
Jackson Memorial Hospital/Ryder
    Trauma Center
and
University of Miami Hospital and Clinics
University of Miami Miller School of
    Medicine
Miami, Florida

John Nagabiez
Department of Surgery
Albany School of Medicine
Albany, New York

Nicholas Namias
Department of Surgery
University of Miami
Coral Gables, Florida

Diego B. Nuñez
Harvard Medical School
and
Neuroradiology and Emergency
    Neuroradiology
Brigham and Women's Hospital
Boston, Massachusetts

Terence O'Keeffe
Division of Trauma, Burns, Critical
    Care and Emergency Surgery
University of Arizona
Tuscon, Arizona

H. Leon Pachter
Department of Surgery
New York University School of Medicine
New York, New York

Hans-Christoph Pape
Department of Trauma
University of Zurich
Zurich, Switzerland

Andrew B. Peitzman
Department of Surgery
University of Pittsburgh School of
    Medicine
Pittsburgh, Pennsylvania

Paul E. Pepe
Department of Emergency Medicine
Southwestern Medical Center
University of Texas
Dallas, Texas

Alan L. Peterson
Department of Psychiatry
Health Science Center
University of Texas at San Antonio
and
Department of Psychology
South Texas Veterans Health Care System
University of Texas at San Antonio
San Antonio, Texas

Mitchell Price
Department of Surgery and Pediatrics
Donald and Barbara Zucker School of
    Medicine at Hofstra/NorthwellHealth
and
Staten Island University Hospital
Staten Island, New York
and
Cohen's Children's Medical Center/
    Northwell Health
East Garden City, New York

Kenneth G. Proctor
Divisions of Trauma and Surgical
    Critical Care
Daughtry Family Department of Surgery
Miller School of Medicine
University of Miami
Miami, Florida

Basil A. Pruitt
Department of Surgery
Uniformed Services University of the
  Health Sciences
Bethesda, Maryland
and
Department of Surgery
UT Health, San Antonio
San Antonio, Texas

Todd E. Rasmussen
Uniformed Services University of the
  Health Sciences
US Air Force
Bethesda, Maryland

Peter Rhee
Grady Memorial Hospital
Department of Surgery at Emory
  Morehouse
Uniformed Services University of the
  Health Sciences
Bethesda, Maryland

Norman Rich
Department of Surgery
Uniformed Services University of the
  Health Science
Walter Reed
Surgery Department
F. Edward Hebert School of Medicine
Bethesda, Maryland

J. David Richardson
Department of Surgery
University of Louisville
Louisville, Kentucky

Ian Roberts
Department of Epidemiology and
  Public Health
Clinical Trials Unit
London, United Kingdom

Michael F. Rotondo
Division of Acute Care Surgery
Department of Surgery
University of Rochester Medical
  Faculty Group
and
Clinical Affairs
University of Rochester Medical Center
Rochester, New York

Grace S. Rozycki
Department of Surgery
The Johns Hopkins University School of
  Medicine
and
Bayview Medical Center
Baltimore, Maryland

Ali Salim
Division of Trauma, Burns, Surgical
Critical Care, and Emergency
Brigham and Women's Hospital
Boston, Massachusetts

Thomas M. Scalea
Department of Surgery
University of Maryland School of
  Medicine
and
R Adams Cowley Shock Trauma Center
  System
University of Maryland Medical System
Baltimore, Maryland

William Schecter
Department of Clinical Surgery
School of Medicine
University of California San Francisco
and
Alliance for Global Clinical Training
Chicago, Illinois

Martin A. Schreiber
Division of Trauma, Critical Care and
    Acute Care Surgery
Department of Surgery
Oregon Health and Science University
Portland, Oregon

Salvatore J.A. Sclafani
Department of Radiology
State University of New York
Downstate Medical School
Brooklyn, New York
and
Azura Vascular Care
Malvern, Pennsylvania

Steven R. Shackford
Department of Surgery
College of Medicine
University of Vermont
Burlington, Vermont

Gerald W. Shaftan
Department of Surgery
Nassau University Medical Center
East Meadow, New York
and
Department of Surgery
State University of New York
Downstate Medical Center
Brooklyn, New York

Ronald Simon
Division of Acute Care Surgery
Department of Surgery
Maimonides Medical Center
Brooklyn, New York

David A. Spain
Division of Acute Care Surgery
Department of Surgery
Stanford University
Stanford, California
and
Trauma Service
Department of Surgery
Stanford Healthcare
Palo Alto, California

H. Harlan Stone
Department of Surgery
University of South Carolina School of
    Medicine Greenville
Greenville, South Carolina

Alex B. Valadka
Department of Neurosurgery
Virginia Commonwealth University
Richmond, Virginia

George C. Velmahos
Department of Surgery
Harvard Medical School
and
Division of Trauma, Emergency Surgery,
    and Surgical Critical Care
Massachusetts General Hospital
Boston, Massachusetts

John A. Weigelt
Department of Surgery
Sanford Health
Sioux Falls, South Dakota
and
Trauma Associates
Lead, South Dakota

Christopher E. White
Trauma and Emergency General Surgery
UT Health San Antonio
San Antonio, Texas

D. Dante Yeh
Ryder Trauma Center
Miami, Florida

CHAPTER 1

Systems of Trauma Care: A Study of Two Counties

West JG, Trunkey DD, Lim RC. Arch Surg 114(4):455–460, 1979

Abstract   Cases of motor vehicle trauma victims, who died after arrival at a hospital, were evaluated in both Orange County (90 cases) and in San Francisco County (92 cases), California. All victims in San Francisco County were brought to a single trauma center, while in Orange County they were transported to the closest receiving hospital. Approximately two-thirds of the non-CNS-related deaths and one-third of the CNS-related deaths in Orange County were judged by the authors as potentially preventable; only one death in San Francisco County was so judged. Trauma victims in Orange County were younger on the average, and the magnitude of their injuries was less than for victims in the San Francisco County. We suggest that survival rates for major trauma can be improved by an organized system of trauma care that includes the resources of a trauma center.

Expert Commentary by Anthony A. Meyer

This landmark paper was a cornerstone in the building of national and international commitment to develop trauma systems to improve care of the injured. This study demonstrated dramatic differences in patient outcomes after motor vehicle crashes in two counties in California: one with an established trauma system (San Francisco County), and one without an effective trauma system (Orange County).

Dr. West was a former resident of both Dr. Trunkey and Dr. Lim. After training, he established a practice in Orange County, California. He was disappointed in the way trauma patients were managed there, compared to his training experience at San Francisco General Hospital (SFGH) where the EMS system in San Francisco brought all trauma victims. He discussed this with Dr. Trunkey and Dr. Lim, two of the attending surgeons at SFGH. Together, they performed this study that got the attention not only of trauma surgeons, but also governmental officials interested in health care.

This study used two relatively new (at that time) methods to study outcomes after motor vehicle crashes (MVC). Injury Severity Scores (ISS) were assigned after review of autopsy records and used to compare actual mortality with the expected mortality at the 50th percentile. Despite having an older, more severely injured patient group, the county with the trauma system had better than expected outcomes, while the county without a trauma system had poorer outcomes.

This study also used an expert panel to review the autopsies of 100 consecutive MVC fatalities that reached a hospital alive. This demonstrated a remarkable difference in the number of preventable, or potentially preventable, deaths of patients in the county without a trauma system, and whether or not death was primarily due to head injury.

The authors acknowledged the limitations of their study; Orange County is seven times larger in size and, at that time, had a somewhat smaller population. However, many subsequent studies have confirmed their findings in other states and other countries by demonstrating the outcome benefits of trauma systems.

This paper provided compelling evidence of the benefit for a coordinated system of trauma care that includes effective EMS transport and expert hospital treatment of the injured. Many subsequent improvements in the management of injured patients are possible because of the existence of the trauma systems that were brought about in part by this study and its authors. Dr. Trunkey, in particular, became a national and international spokesperson and advocate for the development of trauma systems and their benefit to patients everywhere. The magnitude of the impact of this study can't be calculated by an exact measure of avoided death and disability, but it is great and will continue in the future.

Expert Commentary by Frank R. Lewis

This paper was presented before the Western Surgical Association in late 1978 and published in early 1979 in the *Archives of Surgery*. It has probably been more influential in driving the development of regional and statewide trauma systems and individual trauma centers, than any other similar study in the literature; before or since.

In the study, there was a direct comparison of two geographic regions in California (San Francisco and Orange County) with roughly the same population, in the same time frame, one with a single ambulance system and single hospital serving as a trauma center, with comprehensive in-house surgical coverage; the other a dispersed environment with 31 hospitals, and generally only an emergency physician immediately available at night or on weekends.

The numbers of patients studied was small—90 and 92 deaths in the two different regions, respectively—but the authors chose to use preventable death as the outcome measure rather than percentage survival or death in a larger population. This dramatically magnified the difference between the regions. All deaths were autopsied by the local coroner, so cause of death could be accurately identified in all, allowing informed decisions about preventability.

Deaths were classified as central nervous system (CNS)-related or non-CNS-related. In Orange County, there were 60 CNS-related and 30 non-CNS-related deaths. In SF, there were 76 CNS-related and 16 non-CNS-related deaths. Most non-CNS deaths died of hemorrhage, and the judgments in regard to preventability were dramatic:

	Total	Preventable	Possibly Preventable	Non-Preventable	Avg ISS
SF	16	1	0	15	45
OC	30	11	11	8	37

Of the 11 preventable deaths in OC, four were due to a ruptured spleen, four to a lacerated liver, one to perforated small bowel, one to lacerated mesenteric artery, and one due to pericardial tamponade. All deaths occurred more than an hour after hospital arrival, with ample time for operation if facilities had been available, and all were considered surgically controllable. In contrast, the single preventable death in SF was due to late (10 days) aortic rupture in a patient where the chest X-ray did not reveal mediastinal widening; hence no arteriogram was done on presentation. The average ISS was slightly greater in the SF patients and they were mostly over 50, while the OC patients were mostly under 50.

Judgments about preventability were more ambiguous in the CNS deaths, but it was noted that only 12 out of 60 patients in OC received a neurosurgical procedure versus 55 out of 76 in SF, and 8 of the deaths in OC had undiagnosed intracranial hematomas.

Overall, in the non-CNS deaths, 73% of the OC patients were definitely or possibly preventable, while only 7% were so judged in SF. This tenfold difference was so dramatic that it provided a compelling rationale for the expenditure of resources to salvage this mostly young population, who generally could be expected to fully recover and live normally thereafter. Sophisticated or expensive technology was not required; only surgeons and surgical facilities that could provide rapid assessment and competent operative care in a timely manner.

Editor Notes: It is most interesting that such a straightforward analysis as described in this paper could have such a huge impact on the evolution of trauma centers and trauma systems. Ninety trauma deaths in Orange County (OC), where patients were taken to the nearest emergency department, were compared to 92 injury fatalities in San Francisco (SF) County, where a single dedicated trauma center existed, to determine the occurrence of potentially preventable deaths. Among non-CNS-related deaths, only one preventable death was identified in SF County, while 22/30 in Orange County were felt to be clearly or potentially preventable. Furthermore, there were a substantial number of CNS-related deaths in Orange County (28%) judged potentially preventable, possibly related to the lack of aggressive neurosurgical intervention.

Limitations:

Heterogeneity of the population demographics in the two counties may have influenced outcomes;

Transport times may have been substantially longer in the much larger Orange County;

The presence of the medical record in SF may have led to justification of the reason for death, information not always available in Orange County;

Lack of blinding to the county of origin during the analysis may have influenced decision-making.

CHAPTER 2

Relationship between Trauma Center Volume and Outcomes

Nathens AB, Jurkovich GJ, Maier RV, Grossman DC, MacKenzie EJ,
Moore M, Rivara FP. JAMA 285(9):1164–1171, 2001

Abstract　Although this paper is from 2001, there still remains considerable
controversy in 2018 over the volume-outcome relationship, not only in trauma, but
also in surgery in general, particularly regarding oncological and cardiothoracic
procedures. Despite the majority of evidence suggesting that centralization
of care has major advantages, the health care environment still struggles with
this to this day, notably with the advent of for-profit trauma centers in many
states across the nation. Thus, this seminal paper—which was one of the
first and largest to examine whether volume would make a difference where
initial standardization criteria (level designation) had already been met.[1]

Context　The premise underlying regionalization of trauma care is that larger
volumes of trauma patients cared for in fewer institutions will lead to improved
outcomes. However, whether a relationship exists between institutional
volume and trauma outcomes remains unknown.

Objective　To evaluate the association between trauma center volume and
outcomes of trauma patients.

Design　Retrospective cohort study.

Setting　Thirty-one academic level I or level II trauma centers across the United States
participating in the University Health System Consortium Trauma Benchmarking
Study.

Patients　Consecutive patients with penetrating abdominal injury (PAI; n = 478)
discharged between November 1, 1997, and July 31, 1998, or with multisystem
blunt trauma (minimum of head injury and lower-extremity long-bone fractures;
n = 541) discharged between June 1 and December 31, 1998.

Main Outcome Measures　Inpatient mortality and hospital length of stay (LOS),
comparing high-volume (>650 trauma admissions/y) and low-volume
(</= 650 admissions/y) centers.

Results After multivariate adjustment for patient characteristics and injury severity, the relative odds of death were 0.02 (95% confidence interval [CI], 0.002–0.25) for patients with PAI admitted with shock to high-volume centers compared with low-volume centers. No benefit was evident in patients without shock (P = 0.50). The adjusted odds of death in patients with multisystem blunt trauma who presented with coma to a high-volume center was 0.49 (95% CI, 0.26–0.93) versus low-volume centers. No benefit was observed in patients without coma (P = 0.05). Additionally, a shorter LOS was observed in patients with PAI and new Injury Severity Scores (ISS) of 16 or higher (difference in adjusted mean LOS, 1.6 days [95% CI, −1.5–4.7 days]) and in all patients with multisystem blunt trauma admitted to higher-volume centers (difference in adjusted mean LOS, 3.3 days [95% CI, 0.91–5.70 days]).

Conclusions Our results indicate that a strong association exists between trauma center volume and outcomes, with significant improvements in mortality and LOS when volume exceeds 650 cases per year. These benefits are only evident in patients at high risk for adverse outcomes.

Expert Commentary by Lewis Flint

Nathens and coauthors[1] provided data to support one of the basic tenets of design of an effective trauma system: that delivering patients to a center experienced in managing severely injured patients would be associated with improved outcomes (the right patient to the right hospital at the right time). The data were gathered from a recognized national database that was designed to evaluate the effectiveness of trauma centers. The authors selected two categories of patients that would be most likely to show a positive effect of trauma center volume on outcomes: patients with penetrating abdominal injuries with hypovolemic shock and severely injured patients with multisystem blunt force injuries. The data showed that patient volume improved beginning at a level of 650 admissions/year. As with most good surgical research, this report provided insight into an important question and, at the same time, raised other important questions. For example, was volume the important factor or were care processes the vital elements? This intriguing question remains an important consideration. Another question is: does meeting national criteria for trauma center excellence lead to improved outcomes? Data from a national report by MacKenzie and coauthors[2] supported a positive answer. Their data showed that national verification as a trauma center was associated with improved outcomes.

Additional research has provided support for the relationship of increased trauma center patient volume to improved outcomes. Minei and coauthors[3] reported an analysis showing improved injury outcomes with increasing trauma center patient volumes. Similar to the report by Nathens and coauthors[1] the effect was most pronounced in the most severely injured patients. A recent, fascinating report has shown that increased volume leads to improved trauma outcomes but, most important, if volume goes down, the improvement goes away.[4] These observations have important implications for trauma system design.

A final important question raised initially in a 1998 report by Tepas and coauthors[5] relates to the effect of patient volume overload. These data suggested that there was a point at which increasing volume (especially of less severely injured patients) led to diminished outcome quality. This question remains unanswered as do questions regarding the roles of surgeon experience, teamwork, educational commitment, integration of protocols with prehospital care systems, and performance of research in improving patient outcomes. Despite the hallmark article by Nathens and supporting data from other authors we still do not have all the answers we need.

REFERENCES

1. Nathens AB, Jurkovich GJ, Maier RV, Grossman DC, MacKenzie EJ, Moore M, Rivara FP. Relationship between trauma center volume and outcomes. *JAMA*. 2001; 285(9): 1164–1171.
2. MacKenzie EJ, Rivara FP, Jurkovich GJ, Nathens AB, Frey KP, Egleston BL, Salkever DS, Scharfstein DO. A national evaluation of the effect of trauma-center care on mortality. *N Engl J Med*. 2006; 354(4): 366–378.
3. Minei JP, Fabian TC, Guffey DM, Newgard CD, Bulger EM, Brasel KJ, Sperry JL, MacDonald RD. Increased trauma center volume is associated with improved survival after severe injury: Results of a resuscitation outcomes consortium study. *Ann Surg*. 2014; 260(3): 456–464; discussion 464–455.
4. Brown JB, Rosengart MR, Kahn JM, Mohan D, Zuckerbraun BS, Billiar TR, Peitzman AB, Angus DC, Sperry JL. Impact of volume change over time on trauma mortality in the United States. *Ann Surg*. 2017; 266(1): 173–178.
5. Tepas JJ, 3rd, Patel JC, DiScala C, Wears RL, Veldenz HC. Relationship of trauma patient volume to outcome experience: Can a relationship be defined? *J Trauma*. 1998; 44(5): 827–830; discussion 830–821.

Expert Commentary by Terence O'Keeffe

While the study did demonstrate a statistically significant difference between patients treated at a low-volume center (designated as lower than 650 patients/year), it is important to note the absolute numbers involved in some subgroups were small (less than 21). Also, although the database was designed to compare outcomes between trauma centers, not all UHC hospitals contributed to the study, and not all centers contributed to both cohorts, leading to the possibility of bias. Similarly, from personal experience with poor coding of data submitted to the UHC system, I believe that the authors have somewhat downplayed the potential for poor inter-institutional reliability in coding injuries. Sophisticated modeling was employed to examine the volume relationship, but as the authors clearly state, GCS was a critical part of their model and this can often be erroneously measured, especially early in the course of a trauma patient's illness.[1] A follow-up systematic review in 2014 was also somewhat less clear regarding the beneficial effect of trauma volume on outcomes.[2]

However, this push for relentless quality improvement in trauma centers have led many others to examine how we could evaluate metrics among trauma centers to improve benchmarking and decrease complications.[3] From this work and others, the Trauma Quality Improvement Project (TQIP) was born, which aims to further identify best practices among centers and inform individualized performance improvement.[4]

Unfortunately, science has not managed to effect change in the way trauma surgeons would have hoped in the complex health care systems of the twenty-first century, with continued fragmentation of care, multiple states without statewide trauma systems, and competition between centers remaining the order of the day. The call to action in the last paragraph of the manuscript imploring triage of severely injured patients to a few consolidated, dedicated urban trauma centers has been sadly ignored in the scramble for patient volumes and reimbursements. Lack of federal oversight, variations in state designations, and local politics have all contributed to the continuing dearth of regionalization. As an example, a city of 2 million people (Las Vegas) may have only one level I trauma center, whereas another with a population of 3 million (Phoenix) has 11 such centers. This work thus remains as timely today as when it was first published.

REFERENCES

1. Tang A, Pandit V, Fennell V, Jones T, Joseph B, O'Keeffe T, et al. Intracranial pressure monitor in patients with traumatic brain injury. *J Surg Res*. 2015; 194(2): 565–570.
2. Caputo LM, Salottolo KM, Slone DS, Mains CW, Bar-Or D. The relationship between patient volume and mortality in American trauma centres: A systematic review of the evidence. *Injury*. 2014; 45(3): 478–486.
3. Shafi S, Stewart RM, Nathens AB, Friese RS, Frankel H, Gentilello LM. Significant variations in mortality occur at similarly designated trauma centers. *Arch Surg*. 2009; 144(1): 64–68.
4. Shafi S, Nathens AB, Cryer HG, Hemmila MR, Pasquale MD, Clark DE, et al. The trauma quality improvement program of the American College of Surgeons Committee on Trauma. *J Am Coll Surg*. 2009; 209(4): 521–530 e1.

Editor Notes: The impact of trauma centers and patient volume was analyzed in this important paper. Nearly 1,000 patients with either penetrating abdominal injury or multisystem blunt trauma were analyzed for outcomes. High volume centers (those seeing more than 650 cases per year with ISS > 15) had a lower mortality and length of hospital stay in these high-risk trauma patients.

Limitations:

Retrospective study;
Database analysis;
Subset of trauma centers;
Mix of level I and II center data;
Impact of volume on outcome limited to high-risk patients;
Cut point for benefit was derived was arbitrary and derived post hoc.

CHAPTER 3

The Injury Severity Score: A Method for Describing Patients with Multiple Injuries and Evaluating Emergency Care

Baker SP, O'Neill B, Haddon W Jr, Long WB. J Trauma 14(3):187–196, 1974

Abstract Risk estimation for patient prognostication, for individuals and groups, to control for case mix differences in comparative and prospective studies is essential for any public health approach to injury control. It is essential in measuring the impact of primary prevention, secondary prevention (mitigation), and tertiary prevention (treatment).

Author Commentary by Susan P. Baker

In 1970, two years after I received an MPH degree and joined the faculty of the Johns Hopkins School of Public Health, I received a phone call from Dr. William Haddon, president of the Insurance Institute for Highway Safety. He suggested that I tear up the grant proposal I was about to submit to NIH and accept IIHS support for yet-to-be-determined research. That sounded wonderful to me, but the next frustrating months saw a series of my research suggestions rebuffed.

Finally, Haddon and Brian O'Neill, who was then the senior statistician at IIHS and later its president, liked my idea of studying a series of traffic deaths and hospitalized injuries in Baltimore City. We had no inkling that what would evolve would be the ability to measure the effect on trauma survival of having more than one injury. At that time, the Abbreviated Injury Scale (AIS) was the best thing we had for describing injury severity, but it applied only to individual injuries.

In developing my hand-coded form for recording about 2,000 trauma cases (while sitting at my desk in the medical examiner's office, in the days before personal computers), I decided to code not only the most severe injury, as was common practice at the time, but the two injuries with the highest AIS scores. Playing around with the data, I came up with what is a key figure in our paper. I was excited to realize that I had *measured* the influence of additional injuries on the likelihood of death—but everyone I showed it

to said, "Well *of course* it's worse to have more than one injury!"—until
I showed it to Bill Long at a breakfast meeting of trauma docs. Then a young
surgeon at Maryland's "Shock-Trauma Hospital," Bill had been trying to
measure the effects of single-organ and multiple-organ failure. He looked at my
graph for a few moments and said, "This is fascinating—if you square and add
the scores for the two worst injuries, the sum correlates with the case fatality
rate!" As a result, the ISS was conceived. (Subsequently, Brian's analyses showed
it was important to use the three worst injuries rather than just two.)

Forty-three years after publication, the ISS is still valued for its simplicity in
estimating the likelihood of death given a combination of injuries of varied
severity. (The NISS, later developed by Turner Osler, is even simpler and better,
but regrettably is less widely used.)

On a side note, some years ago, a doctor in a novel I was reading—a murder
mystery—exclaimed "Wow! This guy survived with an ISS of 59!" I knew then the
ISS had arrived.

Expert Commentary by Howard R. Champion

In the early 1970s, R.A. Cowley, founder of the University of Maryland Shock
Trauma Unit at Baltimore and the first state-wide trauma system, privately
urged young surgeons, like Bill Long and me, to develop some means of docu-
menting the benefits of his and our endeavors.

Fortunately, our efforts were guided by the knowledge and discipline of Sue
Baker from Johns Hopkins School of Public Health and aided and abetted by
Brian O'Neil and Bill Haddon (of the Haddon Matrix), pioneers in automobile
safety from the Insurance Institute for Highway Safety. Thus, their research created the Injury Severity Score (ISS)—the first and foundational step in developing risk estimates for the anatomic rearrangement complexities that occur
following energy transfer to the human body. In 1974, ISS is described together
with its validation in this seminal paper. It was founded on anatomical descriptors, the Abbreviated Injury Scale (AIS), the development of which was initiated
by aeronautical engineers and has continued to grow over the past five decades
from some 75 injury codes to well over 2,000. Another Johns Hopkins School
of Public Health luminary, Ellen McKenzie, later enabled the use of adminis-
trative databases converting ICD9CM to AIS codes and thus ISS. Meanwhile
we had developed a parallel initiative using ICD8CM to estimate risk based on
analysis of data to create conditional and definitive probabilities of survival, an
approach that was again adopted in the 1990s by Turner Osler.

We also determined that physiological quantifiers as well as the anatomical
description were necessary for accurate risk estimation in the relative minority
of patients who develop acute physiological changes shortly following injury.

Thus, the Triage Index, which was the basis for the Trauma Score and when combined with age and ISS at the Woodstock Conference, produced TRISS— still the most widely used model for controlling for case mix and describing trauma patient populations.[1,2]

As with all advances in science, ISS has been incrementally modified since its visionary creation by Sue Baker, Brian O'Neil, Bill Haddon, and Bill Long. The well-known shortcomings of ISS, including its lack of cross system coherence and wobbly relationship with mortality, have seen many other models created including those for penetrating and combat injury. The methodology for their evaluation has become more disciplined and widespread as has the use of the term "validation."

However, there can be no doubt that the starting point for all of these initiatives was the ISS, developed in the early 1970s. Trauma scoring and risk assessment continue to inspire advanced degree dissertations and research papers. They cross my desk each month from all over the world. They have one thing in common. They all start with ISS.

REFERENCES

1. Champion HR, Copes WS, Sacco WJ, Frey CF, Holcroft JW, et al. Improved predictions from a severity characterization of trauma (ASCOT) over Trauma and Injury Severity Score (TRISS): Results of an independent evaluation. *J Trauma*. 1996; 40(1): 42–48; discussion 48–49.
2. Champion HR, Sacco WJ, Hunt TK. Trauma severity scoring to predict mortality. *World J Surg*. 1983; 7(1): 4–11.

Editor Notes: Prior to this investigation there was no good method of comparing death rates from various medical centers caring for trauma patients. In this paper, the impact of magnitude of injury of a particular body region was classified using data from 128 patients, and then grading was related to mortality. The three most severely injured anatomic body regions were then combined to improve outcome predictions. Today we use Injury Severity Scores (ISS) as a method to help assess how one institution functions when compared to national injury outcomes databases.

Limitations:

Retrospective review without a prospective validation data set;
Limited population size;
Included both penetrating and blunt trauma;
Did not account for multiple injuries in a single anatomic region.

CHAPTER 4

Assessment of Coma and Impaired Consciousness: A Practical Scale

Teasdale G, Jennett B. Lancet 2(7872):81–84, 1974

Abstract   A clinical scale has evolved for assessing the depth and duration of impaired consciousness and coma. Three aspects of behavior are independently measured—motor responsiveness, verbal performance, and eye opening. These can be evaluated consistently by doctors and nurses and recorded on a simple chart, which has proved practical both in a neurosurgical unit and in a general hospital. The scale facilitates consultations between general and special units in cases of recent brain damage and is useful also in defining the duration of prolonged coma.

Expert Commentary by Alex B. Valadka

"Lethargic, obtunded, stuporous, semicomatose"—years ago, a clinician might use such terms to describe the neurological status of an ICU patient. After the physician left the unit, a colleague might choose a different word to characterize the same neurological findings. The patient hadn't changed, but the nursing team was now confused about the patient's status: was he or wasn't he getting better (or worse)?

The Glasgow Coma Scale (GCS) was created to solve this problem. Vague terms were replaced by objective responses. Within the three distinct categories of eye opening, motor response, and verbal response, these objective responses were ranked by correlation with severity of disturbance of consciousness. Charting responses on an ICU flowsheet facilitated immediate visualization of a patient's clinical trajectory. Promptly detecting neurological deterioration by physical findings was especially important because computed tomography had not yet been introduced.

Initially, the GCS used only verbal descriptions. Numerical scores were added later to facilitate entry of grouped data from many patients into computerized databases. For an individual patient, verbal descriptors continue to be preferred.

A particularly useful feature of the GCS is that it is not disease-specific. Its use is appropriate for assessment of impaired consciousness of any etiology. The extent to which it has been widely adopted and modified serves as strong evidence of its universal appeal and ease of use. It soon spread to emergency departments (EDs) for acute assessment of neurologic status. Classification of brain injury as mild, moderate, or severe based on the summed GCS score was described several years after the GCS was introduced.

The GCS has its critics, some of whom point out that it was not created for use in the ED. However, a large body of literature now supports its validity for that application. Others complain that it lacks sensitivity for diagnosing concussion, but the GCS was not developed to be a diagnostic tool for traumatic brain injury. It is meant to measure impairment of consciousness, which is relatively rare in concussed patients. These critics may be using an inappropriate tool to address their needs. Poor inter-rater reliability of GCS assessments and local variations in application and interpretation have also been voiced as concerns, but these are less common when examiners have received proper training in administering and scoring the GCS.

The GCS remains the most widely used assessment tool for acute cerebral disease. The original description of the GCS is among the most highly cited papers in neurosurgery. It helped usher in a new era of assessment, monitoring, and classification of patients with neurological diseases. The 40th anniversary of the description of the GCS occasioned the creation of a website (http://www.glasgowcomascale.org) dedicated to optimizing accurate and reliable use of the GCS.

Timing is everything. An unmet need in the clinical community, a brilliant yet simple idea, and rigorous field-testing of validity all came together to make the description of the GCS one of the most influential clinical neuroscience publications of the past half-century.

Expert Commentary by John C. Marshall

If it can't be expressed in figures, it is not science; it is opinion.

Robert Heinlein

Clinicians rely on numbers to make decisions. We measure the hematocrit to guide transfusion, the diameter of the aorta to guide the management of aneurysms, and the volume of blood loss to inform a decision for thoracotomy. Numbers provide a quantifiable estimate of risk at a point in time and allow us to prognosticate the consequences of a decision. They also provide a tool to measure change over time, and further guide decision-making by defining a trajectory that is either compatible with recovery or grounds for a change in management strategy.

Some phenomena are amenable to measurement using a single variable—the blood glucose level or the oxygen saturation, for example. Others reflecting more complex constructs, such as severity of illness or injury or level of consciousness are not; these latter have stimulated the development of scales or scores to describe the aggregate of a clinical state.

A score is a combination of individual quantitative measures, weighted on the basis of their correlation with an outcome to provide a continuous grade measure of the severity of a clinical state. The advent of the microcomputer and readily accessible software programs to undertake multivariable modeling has resulted in a profusion of scores, robust in their methodology, but of variable clinical utility. Some time-worn scales have persisted, and prominent amongst these is the Glasgow Coma Scale, first proposed by Teasdale and Jennett in 1974[1] and cited almost 12,000 times in the intervening four decades (Google Scholar).

The appeal of the Glasgow Coma Score lies in its simplicity and in its scope. It proceeds from the assumption that altered consciousness is a continuum of abnormality that can change over time, rather than a state that either is or is not present. The Glasgow Coma Score further measures abnormality in three discrete domains—motor responses, verbal responses, and eye opening—and identifies discrete and reproducible abnormalities associated with each level in each domain; for example, flexor versus extensor responses of the limb. It is readily calculated at the bedside and has substantial face validity. It measures those aspects of altered consciousness that the physician recognizes to show graded levels of impairment.

The development of the Glasgow Coma Score was quite informal. Metrics such as positive and negative predictive values or likelihood ratios were not calculated, and inter-observer variability was assessed only in an ad hoc manner. Yet, the tool has become the standard for measuring consciousness following traumatic brain injury, used in a broad spectrum of other neurologic disorders, and has shown good correlation with radiographic, biochemical, and metabolic measures of brain injury.[2] Its limitations notwithstanding, it has become the most widely used tool to measure consciousness and changes in acute neurologic conditions, and, at a population level, to stratify patients for research or guideline development purposes. It is useful for the clinician to understand its original formulation[1] and its reassessment in light of decades of use and advances in the science of acute brain injury.[2]

· REFERENCES

1. Teasdale G, Jennett B. Assessment of coma and impaired consciousness: A practical scale. *Lancet.* 1974; 2: 81–84.
2. Teasdale G, Maas A, Lecky F, Manley G, Stocchetti N, Murray G. The Glasgow Coma Scale at 40 years: Standing the test of time. *Lancet Neurol.* 2014; 13: 844–854.

Editor Notes: The use of the Glasgow Coma Scale (GCS) is widespread in the trauma and critical care world as a means of assessing the level of consciousness. In the original description, a provider disagreement rate of 20% was noted when evaluated impaired cognition. Today, we are aware that the motor score is the clinically relevant aspect of the GCS and is the key element of the score that predicts outcome.

Limitations:

Little data presented;
GCS briefly described but not validated;
Considerable inter-rater variability noted.

CHAPTER 5

The Preventive Treatment of Wound Shock

Cannon WB, Fraser J, Cowell EM. JAMA 70:618–621, 1918

Abstract   This landmark article is one of the most highly referenced papers in modern trauma literatures and lectures. This paper is actually an opinion piece written by Captain Walter B. Cannon, US Army, on treating the combat casualty. He points out the art of trauma surgery advances as a result from lessons learned out of the battlefield. Specifically, reading the paper takes us back to the era of trench warfare in World War I. This paper benefits not only the military trauma surgeon, but everyone who cares for the injured whether it is in the wilderness or the trenches of an inner-city battlefield. This paper presents no data but has a series of vignettes at the end. It describes the casualties and the complex nature of transporting the cold and wet injured through the trenches, which often took hours with a two-man litter-bearing team.

Expert Commentary by David B. Hoyt

Dr. Cannon was deployed as a scientist to study casualties during World War I. This paper describes his observations about principles for treatment of shock.[1] We note that the circumstances he was describing were of trench warfare from the Western Front. At that time, soldiers were deep in narrow trenches connected through a series of passageways to the most forward care—behind the trenches. Carrying a casualty from the forward trench to the first receiving area might occur in darkness, in a very confined space, requiring climbing over and around others in the trench, and take as long as 2 hours to go a short distance. At the time, the theory of shock put forth by Cannon was exemia (where blood and volume were entrapped in a non-circulating vascular bed—as opposed to being shed). Shock was made worse with loss of body heat and acidosis, and treatment was focused on correction of these two factors.

If not attended to and corrected, induction of anesthesia was accompanied with deterioration during operative intervention. His principles for treatment included diligent wrapping of a casualty in multiple blankets with a heating system before transport and delivering warm fluids by mouth.

Because of the known acidosis, delivery of bicarbonate with warm fluids corrected acidosis and was accompanied by restoration of blood pressure in many circumstances with a better outcome. Taken together, warming and correction of acidosis were the standard ways to treat hemorrhagic shock long before replacing fluids as an essential element was realized.

It was in fact not until the 1920s when Blaylock and Harrison performed animal experiments as residents at Vanderbilt that the association between hypovolemia, hypotension, and shock were clearly outlined.[2] These observations were 40 years before the classic experiments of Shires demonstrating the need to resuscitate intercellular swelling and loss of interstitial space fluid while replacing intravascular losses.

The actual use of crystalloid resuscitation was in its infancy during WWI, the first use of intravenous crystalloid dating to the Cholera epidemic in the 1830s.[3] The early delivery of hypertonic crystalloid solutions with added bicarbonate in modest volumes is described in this paper, but it is an afterthought compared to warming and acidosis correction. One of the most important contributions to modern resuscitation was the small comment about "Operative Prophylaxis."

> Injection of a fluid that will increase blood pressure has dangers in itself. Hemorrhage in a case of shock may not have occurred to a marked degree because blood pressure has been too low and the flow too scant to overcome the obstacle offered by a clot. If the pressure is raised before the surgeon is ready to check any bleeding that may take place, blood that is sorely needed may be lost. Fortunately, the injection may be made at the start of operation, just after the patient has been prepared and when the surgeon is ready to stop any hemorrhage, and it may continue as the operation proceeds.

Shaftan affirmed these observations in the 1960s, and Mattox and others emphasized the potential danger with aggressive resuscitation prior to surgical hemostasis in 1994.[4] Vascular surgeons have warned of the danger of bleeding with ruptured aneurysms if blood pressure is restored before surgical control.

"Popping the clot" and increasing bleeding prior to surgical control is now recognized widely. Recent evaluation with a pilot study demonstrated reduced mortality with hypovolemic resuscitation.[5] The use of field tourniquets and pressure dressings—The "Stop the Bleed" program is another recognition of this concept. Cannon's observation in this paper has been relevant for 100 years.

REFERENCES

1. Cannon W, Frawer J, Cowell E. The preventative treatment of wound shock. *JAMA*. 1918; 70: 618–621.
2. Blaylock A. *Principles of Surgical Care in Shock and Other Problems*. CV Mosby Company: St Louis, MO; 1940.
3. Jennings CE. The intra-venous injection of fluid for severe hemorrhage. *Lancet*. 1882; 120: 436–437.
4. Bickell WH, Wall MJ, Pep PE, et al. Immediate versus delayed fluid resuscitation for hypotensive patients with penetrating torso injuries. *N Engl J Med*. 1994; 331: 1105–1109.
5. Schreiber MA, Meier EN, Tisherman SA, et al. A controlled resuscitation strategy is feasible and safe in hypotensive trauma patients: Results of a prospective randomized pilot trial. *J Trauma Acute Care Surg*. 2015; 78: 687–697.

Expert Commentary by Peter Rhee

Dr. Cannon states preferences and beliefs, which have so far withstood time. The introduction is highly profound, obvious and eloquent. Each word is meaningful and insightful. It discusses the importance of the circulatory system, and the ill effects of wound sepsis. The second sentence in the introduction needs to be quoted.

> Everything should be done to promote the factors favorable to restoration of a normal and stable blood flow, and anything unfavorable to such restoration should be scrupulously avoided.

He then reviews two points that are in reference to his previous work and publications: (1) Cooling of a person in shock further lowers blood pressure. (2) Operating on a patient in shock worsens acidosis, which is already present and lowers blood pressure more.

The paper then instructs via detailed specifics how to fold a blanket onto a stretcher and use it to prevent further hypothermia. Because a casualty on the Western Front often passes through the hands of several relays of stretcher bearers and at least three or four medical officers before reaching a clearing station, hypothermia needs to be avoided. Stretcher carrying along trenches may take 1 to 2 hours to get to the regimental aid post. The paper goes on to describe how to make a waterproof sheet-blanket "packet" to be used during stretcher bearing. This packet was to be kept near a fire to keep it warm. This concept of hypothermia prevention was heavily emphasized and used extensively during our most recent conflicts: Operation Enduring Freedom and Operation Iraqi Freedom.

The casualty should be guarded against heat loss, and efficient first aid be given without unduly exposing the patient for long. A hot drink is advised. He also recommends a one-quarter grain of morphine in oral tablet form. For the military surgeon, it is disappointing that our current model of battlefield care is probably not much different than the trench warfare that Dr. Cannon had to experience. It is constantly emphasized that cold, wet clothing, including wet boots, be removed, and the patient covered with pre-warmed wool blankets, offered hot, sweetened alkaline tea, and given a fresh set of hot water bottles. Fast forward 90 years and the military doctrine also adopted the recommendation of oral hydration to combat casualties. This has yet to catch on because of the antiquated recommendation of combat casualties being NPO (nothing by mouth) to appease the anesthesiologists.

Dr. Cannon describes the use of 4% sodium bicarbonate solution that has been warmed. He even points out that if the tube that it has to pass through is of considerable length, recognizing that there is ambient cooling going on, he recommends that the temperature of the fluid be maintained at 110° and 115° F. He then describes how to find and cannulate a vein near the elbow with a hollow needle and to give a pint (473 cc) over 15–20 minutes by holding the fluid 2–3 feet above the patient.

Because acidosis and hypotension interact and contribute to the development of each other, emphasis is again placed on resuscitation with oral bicarbonate solutions. The paper then goes into several vignettes to prove his beliefs. "German officer wounded in the buttocks with hypotension (78/56) and oral bicarb therapy started. Second day the wounds were evidently infected with gas but the blood pressure was better at 102/66. In spite of operation, the infection spread and death resulted."

He states that the fluids are lost from the circulation, and the blood becomes stagnant and concentrated. Normal saline or Ringer's solution fails to combat acidosis and actually increases an already existent acidosis. After much emphasis for the use of bicarbonate injections to treat acidosis (including intrarectal injections), he states the following:

> injection of a fluid that will increase blood pressure has dangers itself.... If the pressure is raised before the surgeon is ready to check any bleeding that may take place, blood that is sorely needed may be lost.

This previous statement has been repeatedly quoted by experts on trauma.

The rest of the paper is a short description of five more casualties and the effects of surgery and the bicarbonate solutions. Reading of these soldiers and their injuries are precious for the battlefield surgeon. Of note was that most of the surgery was not immediate but days later after resuscitation with the bicarbonate injections. Thus, the emphasis on oral hydration with alkaline tea. There are many things to take away from this paper including an understanding of the knowledge of physiology and hemorrhagic shock. However, the common-sense observations are precious including specific methodology of keeping a patient warm. It emphasizes the commonsense wisdom of being able to balance the Yin and Yang of hemorrhage source control, while keeping the patient alive with resuscitation. As we learn and relearn physiology, it should be noted that it wasn't long ago when we emphasized resuscitation with crystalloid solutions as a priority before hemorrhage source control.

It is only now that we are also learning the concept that blood and crystalloids are vastly different. We should, however, continue to investigate the development of resuscitation fluid that has buffering capacity with alkaline components. This paper is a joy to digest and is highly recommended by all trauma surgeons.

Editor Notes: This classic paper by Cannon and colleagues during World War I stressed the need to avoid hypothermia or operative intervention in patients in shock. In fact, half of the article focuses on how to keep a patient warm and dry during transport to medical care. Some prescient observations were made by these astute clinicians: "Injection of a fluid that will increase blood pressure has dangers in itself. Hemorrhage in the case of shock may not have occurred to a marked degree because blood pressure has been too low and the flow too scant to overcome the obstacle offered by a clot. If the pressure is raised before the surgeon is ready to check any bleeding that may take place; blood that is sorely needed may be lost."

Limitations:

The paper is a set of recommendations based on the observations of three physicians in combat hospitals during WWI;
Only case examples are given for the recommendations;
No data was analyzed.

CHAPTER 6

Immediate versus Delayed Fluid Resuscitation for Hypotensive Patients with Penetrating Torso Injuries

Bickell WH, Wall MJ Jr, Pepe PE, Martin RR, Ginger VF, Allen MK, Mattox KL. N Engl J Med 331(17):1105–1109, 1994

Abstract The "scoop and run" concept for prehospital care was introduced in 1982,[1] but it is often attributed to the landmark paper by Bickell et al. 12 years later.[2] The prehospital care of trauma victims follows either one of two fundamentally different management principles. The first involves stabilizing the patient with as much medical care and fluid as necessary at the scene, and is typical throughout Europe. The "scoop and run" concept involves providing only basic life support in the field, with minimal fluid resuscitation, and immediate transport. This is typical throughout North America and can be directly attributed to Bickell et al.[2]

Background Fluid resuscitation may be detrimental when given before bleeding is controlled in patients with trauma. The purpose of this study was to determine the effects of delaying fluid resuscitation until the time of operative intervention in hypotensive patients with penetrating injuries to the torso.

Methods We conducted a prospective trial comparing immediate and delayed fluid resuscitation in 598 adults with penetrating torso injuries who presented with a prehospital systolic blood pressure of < or = 90 mmHg. The study setting was a city with a single centralized system of prehospital emergency care and a single receiving facility for patients with major trauma. Patients assigned to the immediate-resuscitation group received standard fluid resuscitation before they reached the hospital and in the trauma center, and those assigned to the delayed-resuscitation group received intravenous cannulation but no fluid resuscitation until they reached the operating room.

Results Among the 289 patients who received delayed fluid resuscitation, 203 (70%) survived and were discharged from the hospital, as compared with 193 of the 309 patients (62%) who received immediate fluid resuscitation (P = 0.04). The mean estimated intraoperative blood loss was similar in the two groups. Among the 238 patients in the delayed-resuscitation group who survived to the postoperative period, 55 (23%) had one or more complications (adult respiratory distress syndrome, sepsis syndrome, acute renal failure,

coagulopathy, wound infection, and pneumonia), as compared with 69 of
the 227 patients (30%) in the immediate-resuscitation group (P = 0.08).
The duration of hospitalization was shorter in the delayed-resuscitation group.

Conclusions   For hypotensive patients with penetrating torso injuries, delay of
aggressive fluid resuscitation until operative intervention improves the outcome.

Author Commentary by Paul E. Pepe

In 1982, standard textbook practice was to purposely raise systemic blood pressure (SBP) for hypotensive trauma patients with presumed internal hemorrhage
using the pneumatic anti-shock garment (PASG) and large-scale intravenous
(IV) infusions of isotonic fluids. However, to justify PASG application in our
own EMS system (Houston, TX), we first implemented a clinical trial.

Unexpectedly, we found *worse* outcomes, even in patients with penetrating
abdominal injuries for whom a presumed tamponade effect of the PASG was
considered an added advantage. The worse outcome was a somewhat surprising
result. Control and study groups were well-matched, and SBP was raised significantly as intended. Speculations were made, but, initially, we just dismissed the
PASG as offering no demonstrable advantage. But this also opened us to new
considerations.

In one of several exemplary index cases, a young man arrived at our trauma
center one day with an accidentally amputated arm. Reportedly, he hemor-
rhaged significantly on-site and during direct transport in a private automobile
from that nearby scene. Though hypotensive/tachycardic upon arrival, he was
relatively alert. Much of the bleeding had stopped, presumably due to arterial spasm. Shortly after infusing a large volume of IV fluids (per standard of
care), the wound suddenly re-bled quite significantly. We rapidly controlled that
extremity hemorrhage and reconfirmed "successful" blood pressure restoration
to "normal" levels. But we also reflected that the "therapy" had also re-induced
the bleeding.

Among other experiences being discussed by my very wise senior surgical
co-investigators, including the eminent Dr. Kenneth Mattox, such observations
begged the question: "Does immediately infusing fluids to patients with internal
bleeding have the same detrimental effect, but one we cannot directly observe?"
Multidisciplinary practitioners had always been hesitant about fluid infusions
in aortic dissection and gastrointestinal bleeding. Why was this any different?

Now re-examining the PASG data, it appeared, retrospectively, the worse
outcomes were clearly related to cases in which there was a distinct primary

vascular injury. Also, a more in-depth review of "classic" literature (e.g., from World War I) revealed that this was not at all a new observation. Many others had published similar concerns. The 1970s–1980s rationale for fluid infusions to elevate SBP had emanated out of elegant animal experiments conducted in the mid-twentieth century. These demonstrated the clear value of that intervention—but only when used as a restorative treatment *after the bleeding had already been controlled.*

Our most brilliant fellow, Dr. Bill Bickell, who we had borrowed from the military to lead the PASG studies, soon conducted vanguard laboratory studies of infusing fluids in *uncontrolled hemorrhage models*, demonstrating hydrostatic acceleration of hemorrhage, dislodgement of soft clots, and dilution of clotting factors. Our resulting clinical trial involving hypotensive patients with penetrating truncal trauma (the 1994 publication cited here) did indeed demonstrate worse outcomes with early fluid resuscitation. Unfortunately, those findings were not yet ready for "prime time" acceptance. Several decades later, however, investigations into damage control resuscitation help to further explain our findings and also provide reassurances that we were fortuitously on the right track at the time.

Expert Commentary by Kenneth G. Proctor

In 598 hypotensive adults with penetrating torso trauma, Bickell et al. reported[2] that 289 patients were randomized to receive delayed fluid resuscitation, and 203 (70%) survived to hospital discharge, compared with 193 of the 309 patients (62%) randomized to immediate fluid resuscitation (P = 0.04). This finding challenged traditional wisdom about early large volume resuscitation of hemorrhagic shock, but was supported by extensive pre-clinical work,[3-6] which clearly showed detrimental effects of isotonic normal saline (NS) or lactated Ringers (LR) and, in turn, reinvigorated interest in the use of low-volume alternatives, such as hypertonic saline (HS) ± dextran (D).

An initial prehospital randomized controlled trial (RCT) reported that HSD patients required less fluid and arrived with higher SBP than patients receiving LR. Survival was improved, especially in those with head injury.[7] Additional RCTs rapidly followed,[8,9] affirming the benefits of small volume HS, relative to either LR or NS, especially in those with low Glasgow Coma Score (GCS), in terms of SBP on admission and survival, but no added benefit of D. The exact explanation remained elusive until Rhee et al. in 2000 reported that various (supposedly) "pharmacologically inert" saline resuscitation solutions with or without colloids, in fact, caused dose-related increases in human neutrophil activation and adhesion in vitro.[10] Regardless, by 2006, at least 32 RCTs in 8,452 critically ill patients found no evidence that added albumin decreased mortality relative to crystalloid alone.[11] By 2007, there were at least 55 RCTs in 7,754 patients who showed no evidence that any colloid decreased mortality relative to crystalloid alone.[12] By 2008, there were at least 70 RCTs in 4,375 patients who showed no evidence that any one colloid was safer or more effective than another.[13] Nevertheless, in the subset of patients with severe traumatic brain injury, prehospital resuscitation with HSD generally modulates inflammatory, coagulation, and endothelial activation marker profiles,[14] and that either HS or HSD specifically attenuates activation and promotes apoptosis of neutrophils.[15] Thus, by 2010, most were convinced that prehospital HS or HSD, relative to LR or NS, restores cerebral perfusion, reduces cerebral edema and modulates inflammation, to reduce secondary neuronal injury after traumatic brain injury. Unfortunately, the data didn't agree; a double-blind, placebo-controlled RCT involving 114 North American emergency medical service agencies within the Resuscitation Outcomes Consortium was terminated early for futility when a 6-month neurologic outcome was no different in head-injured patients who received a single 250 mL bolus of HSD, HS, or NS.[16]

Anticipating improved mortality, many trauma systems adopted the concept of restricted prehospital fluid suggested by Bickell et al.[2] Unfortunately, that reality also does not exactly conform to the theory. In 2000, a European study found that intentionally withholding fluids until hospital arrival had no mortality benefit.[17] In 2002, Dutton et al. reported no difference in mortality with target mean arterial pressure (MAP) of 100 and 70 mmHg.[18] In 2011, several investigators from Bickell's original group observed no mortality benefit with a fluid resuscitation target MAP of 50 versus 65 mmHg.[19] Five years later, the same group randomized penetrating trauma patients with SBP <90 mmHg requiring emergent laparotomy or thoracotomy to a target MAP of either 65 or 50 mmHg. That study was terminated early with no difference in 30-day mortality.[20] Carrick et al. followed with a review of five RCTs, including the original Bickell et al. study, to examine the value of hypotensive resuscitation or permissive hypotension until bleeding is operatively controlled. They concluded that aggressive prehospital or hospital fluid resuscitation leads to more complications than hypotensive resuscitation, but there was no survival benefit.[21] Since the populations, timing of interventions, and outcomes studied in each RCT were slightly different, they concluded that only a large, multicenter RCT can unequivocally establish the benefit of hypotensive resuscitation after trauma.

Thus, more than 20 years ago, the study by Bickell et al. ignited a firestorm of investigations that continues today. The current thinking is that there is no categorical evidence either for or against early or large-volume fluid administration and continued uncertainty about the best fluid or optimal target for bleeding trauma patients.[22]

REFERENCES

1. Gervin AS, Fischer RP. The importance of prompt transport of salvage of patients with penetrating heart wounds. *J Trauma*. 1982; 22(6): 443–448.
2. Bickell WH, Wall MJ Jr, Pepe PE, Martin RR, Ginger VF, Allen MK, Mattox KL. Immediate versus delayed fluid resuscitation for hypotensive patients with penetrating torso injuries. *New Engl J Med*. 1994; 331(17): 1105–1109.
3. Bickell WH, Bruttig SP, Millnamow GA, O'Benar J, Wade CE. The detrimental effects of intravenous crystalloid after aortotomy in swine. *Surgery*. 1991; 110(3): 529–536.
4. Bickell WH, Bruttig SP, Millnamow GA, O'Benar J, Wade CE. Use of hypertonic saline/dextran versus lactated Ringer's solution as a resuscitation fluid after uncontrolled aortic hemorrhage in anesthetized swine. *Ann Emerg Med*. 1992; 21(9): 1077–1085.
5. Shaftan GW, Chiu CJ, Dennis C, Harris B. Fundamentals of physiologic control of arterial hemorrhage. *Surgery*. 1965; 58(5): 851–856.
6. Sondeen JL, Coppes VG, Holcomb JB. Blood pressure at which rebleeding occurs after resuscitation in swine with aortic injury. *J Trauma*. 2003; 54(5 Suppl): S110–S117.
7. Vassar MJ, Perry CA, Gannaway WL, Holcroft JW. 7.5% sodium chloride/dextran for resuscitation of trauma patients undergoing helicopter transport. *Arch Surg*. 1991; 126(9): 1065–1072.
8. Vassar MJ, Fischer RP, O'Brien PE, Bachulis BL, Chambers JA, Hoyt DB, Holcroft JW. A multicenter trial for resuscitation of injured patients with 7.5% sodium chloride: The effect of added dextran 70—The multicenter group for the study of hypertonic saline in trauma patients. *Arch Surg*. 1993; 128(9): 1003–1011; discussion 1011–1013.
9. Vassar MJ, Perry CA, Holcroft JW. Prehospital resuscitation of hypotensive trauma patients with 7.5% NaCl versus 7.5% NaCl with added dextran: A controlled trial. *J Trauma*. 1993; 34(5): 622–632; discussion 632–633.
10. Rhee P, Wang D, Ruff P, Austin B, DeBraux S, Wolcott K, Burris D, Ling G, Sun L. Human neutrophil activation and increased adhesion by various resuscitation fluids. *Crit Care Med*. 2000; 28(1): 74–78.
11. Liberati A, Moja L, Moschetti I, Gensini GF, Gusinu R. Human albumin solution for resuscitation and volume expansion in critically ill patients. *Intern Emerg Med*. 2006; 1(3): 243–245.
12. Perel P, Roberts I. Colloids versus crystalloids for fluid resuscitation in critically ill patients. *Cochrane Database Syst Rev*. 2007; 105(4): CD000567. Update in: *Cochrane Database Syst Rev*. 2011; 3(3): CD000567.
13. Bunn F, Trivedi D, Ashraf S. Colloid solutions for fluid resuscitation. *Cochrane Database Syst Rev*. 2008; (1): CD001319. Update in: *Cochrane Database Syst Rev*. 2011; (3): CD001319.
14. Rhind SG, Crnko NT, Baker AJ, Morrison LJ, Shek PN, Scarpelini S, Rizoli SB. Prehospital resuscitation with hypertonic saline-dextran modulates inflammatory, coagulation and endothelial activation marker profiles in severe traumatic brain injured patients. *J Neuroinflammation*. 2010; 7: 5.
15. Junger WG, Rhind SG, Rizoli SB, Cuschieri J, Baker AJ, Shek PN, Hoyt DB, Bulger EM. Prehospital hypertonic saline resuscitation attenuates the activation and promotes apoptosis of neutrophils in patients with severe traumatic brain injury. *Shock*. 2013; 40(5): 366–374.

16. Bulger EM, May S, Brasel KJ, Schreiber M, Kerby JD, Tisherman SA, Newgard C, et al. ROC Investigators: Out-of-hospital hypertonic resuscitation following severe traumatic brain injury—A randomized controlled trial. *JAMA*. 2010; 304(13): 1455–1464.

17. Turner J, Nicholl J, Webber L, Cox H, Dixon S, Yates D. A randomised controlled trial of prehospital intravenous fluid replacement therapy in serious trauma. *Health Technol Assess*. 2000; 4(31): 1–57.

18. Dutton RP, Mackenzie CF, Scalea TM. Hypotensive resuscitation during active hemorrhage: Impact on in-hospital mortality. *J Trauma*. 2002; 52(6): 1141–1146.

19. Morrison CA, Carrick MM, Norman MA, Scott BG, Welsh FJ, Tsai P, Liscum KR, Wall MJ Jr, Mattox KL. Hypotensive resuscitation strategy reduces transfusion requirements and severe postoperative coagulopathy in trauma patients with hemorrhagic shock: Preliminary results of a randomized controlled trial. *J Trauma*. 2011; 70(3): 652–663.

20. Carrick MM, Morrison CA, Tapia NM, Leonard J, Suliburk JW, Norman MA, Welsh FJ, et al. Intraoperative hypotensive resuscitation for patients undergoing laparotomy or thoracotomy for trauma: Early termination of a randomized prospective clinical trial. *J Trauma Acute Care Surg*. 2016; 80(6): 886–896.

21. Carrick MM, Leonard J, Slone DS, Mains CW, Bar-Or D. Hypotensive resuscitation among trauma patients. *BioMed Res Int*. 2016; 2016: 8901938.

22. Cotton BA, Jerome R, Collier BR, Khetarpal S, Holevar M, Tucker B, Kurek S, et al. Eastern association for the surgery of trauma practice parameter workgroup for prehospital fluid resuscitation: Guidelines for prehospital fluid resuscitation in the injured patient. *J Trauma*. 2009; 67(2): 389–402.

Editor Notes: This was an extremely important paper that brought to our attention the potential dangers of aggressive fluid resuscitation. Among 598 hypotensive patients with penetrating torso injuries, those receiving fluids in the field had a higher mortality than those where fluid administration was restricted until reaching the operating room (mortality 38% vs. 30%, P - 0.04).

Limitations:

Alternate day group inclusion (not a randomized trial);
Single city experience;
Limited to penetrating trauma;
Crossover occurred in the delayed-resuscitation group accidentally or when deemed necessary (8%);
As there was only an absolute difference in mortality of just 10 patients, crossover to receive fluids in 22 patients in the delayed group may have influenced survival;
There were no statistically significant differences in complications.

CHAPTER 7

Effects of Tranexamic Acid on Death, Vascular Occlusive Events, and Blood Transfusion in Trauma Patients with Significant Hemorrhage (CRASH-2): A Randomized, Placebo-Controlled Trial

CRASH-2 Trial Collaborators, Shakur H, Roberts I, et al. Lancet 376(9734):23–32, 2010

Abstract   This important paper addressed a key clinical question, which was exceptionally novel at the time of investigation. Namely, could the early administration of 1 gram of tranexamic acid (TXA) administered over 10 minutes (as a loading dose) followed by a 1 gram infusion over the subsequent 8 hours improve key outcomes compared to placebo in trauma victims deemed at risk for significant bleeding?

Background   Tranexamic acid can reduce bleeding in patients undergoing elective surgery. We assessed the effects of early administration of a short course of tranexamic acid on death, vascular occlusive events, and the receipt of blood transfusion in trauma patients.

Methods   This randomized controlled trial was undertaken in 274 hospitals in 40 countries. 20,211 adult trauma patients with, or at risk of, significant bleeding were randomly assigned within 8 hours of injury to either tranexamic acid (loading dose 1 gram over 10 minutes then infusion of 1 gram over 8 hours) or matching placebo. Randomization was balanced by center, with an allocation sequence based on a block size of eight, generated with a computer random number generator. Both participants and study staff (site investigators and trial coordinating center staff) were masked to treatment allocation. The primary outcome was death in the hospital within 4 weeks of injury, and was described with the following categories: bleeding, vascular occlusion (myocardial infarction, stroke, and pulmonary embolism), multiorgan failure, head injury, and other. All analyses were by intention to treat. This study is registered as ISRCTN86750102 clinicaltrials.gov NCT00375258 and South African Clinical Trial Register DOH-27-0607-1919.

Findings   10,096 patients were allocated to tranexamic acid, and 10,115 to placebo, of whom 10,060 and 10,067, respectively, were analyzed. All-cause mortality was significantly reduced with tranexamic acid (1463 [14.5%] tranexamic acid group vs. 1613 [16.0%] placebo group; relative risk 0.91, 95% CI 0.85–0.97; p = 0.0035). The risk of death due to bleeding was significantly reduced (489 [4.9%] vs. 574 [5.7%]; relative risk 0.85, 95% CI 0.76–0.96; p = 0.0077).

Interpretation   Tranexamic acid safely reduced the risk of death in bleeding trauma patients in this study. On the basis of these results, tranexamic acid should be considered for use in bleeding trauma patients.

Funding   UK NIHR Health Technology Assessment programme, Pfizer, BUPA Foundation, and JP Moulton Charitable Foundation.

Author Commentary by Ian Roberts

Worldwide, traumatic bleeding kills around 2 million people each year, with over 90% of the deaths in low- and middle-income countries. Tranexamic acid (TXA) is an antifibrinolytic drug that has been licensed for use for many years to treat heavy menstrual periods and for dental extraction in people with bleeding disorders. It was also sporadically used to reduce blood transfusion in surgical patients.

The seed that became the CRASH-2 trial was planted in 2006, when I read the results of a systematic review of randomized trials of antifibrinolytic drugs in elective surgery. Antifibrinolytics (aprotinin or TXA) reduced the need for blood transfusion by one-third, reduced donor exposure by one unit, and halved the need for further surgery to control bleeding. The differences were all highly statistically significant. There was also a statistically non-significant reduction in the risk of death in the antifibrinolytic treated group.

Since being cut open by a surgeon and being slashed by a machete are not completely different from a hemostatic viewpoint, we thought that TXA had the potential to reduce mortality in bleeding trauma patients. We searched the literature to see if such a trial had already been done but there was nothing at all. I had been searching for a potential intervention to reduce bleeding deaths for a long time, and this looked like a winner.

At that time, there was a lot of interest in hemostatic drugs because Novo Nordisk were pushing recombinant activated factor seven. We had just finished the CRASH trial of corticosteroids in traumatic brain injury (10,000 patients) and had built up a large global network of collaborating centers. We realized that we could build on this network to conduct a large trial of tranexamic acid in acute traumatic bleeding.

We started the trial with very little funding but eventually managed to get funding support from the UK National Institute for Health Research (NIHR). The trial required a huge effort from hundreds of doctors and nurses around the world, but it was worth it. A total of 20,211 patients were recruited from 274 hospitals in 40 countries.

The results showed that TXA reduces mortality with no apparent increase in side effects. If given promptly, TXA reduces the risk of bleeding to death by about a third. On the basis of these results, it has been estimated that giving TXA to bleeding trauma patients could save up to 200,000 lives per year worldwide. Analysis showed that TXA administration is highly cost effective in high-, middle-, or low-income countries. On the basis of the trial results, tranexamic acid was included on the World Heath Organization (WHO) List of Essential Medicines and incorporated into trauma treatment guidelines in many countries.

Tranexamic acid is a cheap generic drug but has huge potential to save lives. We are fortunate to live in a country where you can obtain public funds for patient centered research, despite there being little commercial interest from the pharmaceutical industry.

Expert Commentary by Joseph J. DuBose

The potential benefit of tranexamic acid in this setting was based upon previous experience in patients with bleeding risk in select surgical arenas—including the realms of cardiac surgery, neurosurgery, and orthopedic surgery. These cumulative experiences had demonstrated the relative safety and cost effectiveness of this pharmacologic adjunct.

The study itself was a very large undertaking, including 20,211 patients admitted to 274 hospitals in 40 countries across six continents. While this produced a broad sample, it proved noteworthy that less than 2% of patients were recruited from countries with the most significant investment in trauma systems—such as the United States, Canada, the United Kingdom, or Western European nations. The relative paucity of patients from these regions—where access to early intervention and blood for resuscitation are more common—proved a criticism of the effort.

Other elements of this investigation have also received criticism. Trauma patients were enrolled if they were deemed to be "at high risk of bleeding." This was defined as being indicated by as little as a single systolic blood pressure after injury of less than 100 mmHg or a heart rate of more than 100 beats per minute—neither of which is particularly specific for bleeding. In addition, they did not assess clinically relevant mechanisms and relied on clinical impression for such complications as venous thrombosis. Finally, while conceptualized as a study to assess the hemostatic effects of tranexamic acid, the achieved patient enrollment resulted in a large worldwide cohort of variably injured patients with varying blood loss and requirements for interventions.

Despite these challenges, the sheer size of the obtained cohort and the results of this work are impossible to dismiss. The relative risk (RR) of death in the TXA group was 0.91 (95% CI 0.85–0.97), without significant increase in vascular occlusive events. Mortality was reduced from 16.0% to 14.5% (RR 0.91, 95% CI 0.85–0.97, p = 0.0035). Although the treatment and control groups had similar transfusion requirements, the absolute risk reduction for mortality with TXA use was 5.7% compared to 4.9% for the placebo arm. A subsequent analysis would demonstrate that the greatest benefit was achieved among patients administered TXA less than 3 hours after injury—a concern that should be noted by all when considering TXA use.

Based upon this landmark paper, TXA has now become a part of massive transfusion protocols at many leading trauma centers throughout the world. The topic of TXA use in trauma remains an active area of investigation, with recent work focusing on better defining the action of TXA and optimal selection of patients for this adjunct using thromboelastography and other adjuncts.

Editor Notes: This huge clinical trial compared the use of tranexamic acid (TXA) to placebo for the care of trauma patients with hemorrhage. Risk of death was reduced in the TXA study, as was death due to bleeding. Because TXA has an extensive track record for safety and is very low cost, this paper led to widespread implementation of the drug in the setting of massive transfusion, despite a number of methodological concerns.

Limitations:

Most of the patients in this study were not experiencing hemorrhage (50% did not receive transfusions);

Many of the patients were accrued from facilities in developing nations where prehospital care and rapidity of transport to the hospital are variable;

Penetrating mechanism was high (1/3);

Patients were generally young (75% < 45 years), and minimally deranged physiologically (70% with a normal systolic BP, 2/3 had GCS > 12, and half had a normal heart rate);

Accrual of patients occurred over a long period of time (5 years);

The nearly 100% compliance in patient follow-up that is reported, appears unlikely;

And finally, the mortality was actually greater with TXA administered more than 3 hours after injury.

CHAPTER 8

Base Deficit as a Guide to Volume Resuscitation

Davis JW, Shackford SR, Mackersie RC, Hoyt DB. J Trauma 28(10):1464–1467, 1988

Abstract   The base deficit (BD) is a potentially useful indicator of volume deficit in trauma patients. To evaluate BD as an index for fluid resuscitation, the records of 209 trauma patients with serial arterial blood gases (ABG) were reviewed. The patients were grouped according to initial BD: mild, 2 to −5; moderate, −6 to −14; and severe, < −15. The volume of resuscitative fluid administered, change in BD, mean arterial pressure (MAP), and presence of ongoing hemorrhage were analyzed for differences between the BD groups.

The MAP decreased significantly, and the volume of fluid required for resuscitation increased with increasing severity of BD group. A BD that increased (became more negative) with resuscitation was associated with ongoing hemorrhage in 65%. The data suggest that the BD is a useful guide to volume replacement in the resuscitation of trauma patients.

Author Commentary by James W. Davis

The determination of the end points of resuscitation using vital signs is not reliable. Biochemical indicators of shock and the efficacy of resuscitation have been sought, and remain, somewhat elusive. Excess lactate had been described as a marker of anaerobic metabolism and oxygen debt but was not readily available, and there was no point of care testing. In a 1969 study from the Da Nang Navy Medical Center, Base Deficit (BD) was a better determinate than pH of resuscitation from shock after 24 hours. BD was described as "nearly stoichiometric with lactate" in a review article published in *Surgical Clinics of North America* in 1982.

There was a strong influence from the Navy experience in Vietnam and the Division of Trauma at the University of California, San Diego Division. An arterial blood gas (which included BD) was part of the admission trauma laboratory panel when I arrived as the trauma fellow in 1987, but there was no data on the use of BD in active resuscitation. This became the catalyst for this research project.

This study included 209 blunt and penetrating trauma patients. The BD values were collected and categorized. BD categories were initially defined as mild

(2 to −5), moderate (−6 to −14), and severe (≤ −15). The data demonstrated that with worsening BD, patients had lower initial systolic blood pressure, increased fluid and transfusion requirements, and increased injury severity score (ISS) mortality. This study also demonstrated that the base deficit improved rapidly in most patients with resuscitation and that a base deficit that did improve, in spite of resuscitation, was an indicator of ongoing hemorrhage. These categories were refined in 1996 and in other studies to include normal (2 to −2), mild (−3 to −5), moderate (−6 to −9), and severe (≤ −10).

There have been numerous subsequent publications establishing the use of BD as a biochemical marker of shock, mortality, and resuscitation. A BD ≤ −6 has been repeatedly shown to identify trauma patients at high risk for mortality and the need for transfusion.

Expert Commentary by Raul Coimbra

The seminal work by Davis et al., presented at the Western Trauma Association and published in *The Journal of Trauma* in 1988, marked a new era in trauma resuscitation. Taken for granted today, the concept of using a serum biomarker to guide volume resuscitation and assess adequacy of resuscitation and bleeding control was critically important in the management of severely injured patients at the time. The authors grouped trauma patients according to initial base deficit levels; mild: +2 to −5; moderate: −6 to −14; and severe: < −15. As mean arterial pressure decreased and fluid requirements increased, BD increased. They found that an increase in BD during ongoing resuscitation was associated with continued hemorrhage in 65% of the patients and concluded that base deficit should be used as a guide to volume replacement. The importance is such, that 30 years later, serum biomarkers, such as BD and lactate, remain as critical data elements in the assessment of tissue perfusion and oxygen debt.

Shock is defined as circulatory dysfunction causing decreased tissue oxygenation and accumulation of oxygen debt, which can ultimately lead to multiorgan system failure. In the multiple trauma victim, shock generally occurs due to hypovolemia from acute blood loss, making the assessment of hemodynamic status and perfusion a key principle in the resuscitation phase. Subsequent monitoring to screen for ongoing hemorrhage and to assess the efficacy of resuscitation is vital in avoiding preventable death and significant morbidity in these patients. Therefore, resuscitation strategies should optimize tissue perfusion while avoiding complications of overaggressive volume replacement, such as the exacerbation of hemorrhage, pulmonary edema, and intracranial hypertension following brain injury.

Since the work of Davis et al., the measurement of serum lactate has become more ubiquitous, cheap, easy to perform, and to some extent, it has replaced base deficit as a marker of oxygen debt, particularly because of its potential deployment in the prehospital setting. In addition, many other techniques have been developed and used without much success. Examples include near infrared spectroscopy, side stream dark field video microscopy, and sublingual or gastric capnometry, just to name a few. These techniques are limited in its clinical applicability, are high cost, require training, and its reliability in different clinical scenarios has been questioned.

There are several strategies to diagnose shock and monitor volume resuscitation in hemorrhaging trauma patients, including hemodynamic monitoring and measurement of global and tissue-specific perfusion. Some of these techniques are highly invasive and impractical in the acute resuscitation phase. Other less-invasive techniques, such as tissue pO_2, pCO_2, and pH measurements and thoracic electrical bioimpedance, are not well studied but may offer viable alternatives in the future.

As suggested by Davis et al., serum markers of shock, such as BD and serum lactate, provide a rapid assessment of tissue oxygen debt and volume resuscitation requirements. In addition, they also suggest ongoing hemorrhage when the values "do not move in the right direction" toward normalcy, but pressures are in the normal range during initial resuscitation.

SUGGESTED REFERENCES

Davis JW, Shackford SR, Mackersie RC, Hoyt DB. Base deficit as a guide to volume resuscitation. *J Trauma*. 1988; 28: 1464–1467.

Englehart MS, Schreiber MA. Measurement of acid–base resuscitation endpoints: Lactate, base deficit, bicarbonate or what? *Curr Opin Crit Care* 2006; 12: 569–574.

Holley A, Lukin W, Paratz J, Hawkins T, Boots R, Lipman J. Review article: Part one: Goal-directed resuscitation – Which goals? Haemodynamic targets. *EMA* 2012; 24: 14–22.

Holley A, Lukin W, Paratz J, Hawkins T, Boots R, Lipman J. Review article: Part two: Goal-directed resuscitation – Which goals? Perfusion targets. *EMA* 2012; 1: 127–135.

Wilson M, Davis DP, Coimbra R. Diagnosis and monitoring of hemorrhagic shock during the initial resuscitation of multiple trauma patients: A review. *J Emerg Med*. 2003; 24: 413–422.

Editor Notes: The authors analyzed patients who presented to their trauma center with hypotension and demonstrated that base deficit was a valuable guide for resuscitation. Patients with greater BD clearly received more aggressive fluid resuscitation in the authors' institution. Furthermore, as patients were resuscitated, the change in base deficit diminished, suggesting a decrease in the need for resuscitation.

Limitations:

Base deficit examined only in patients with hypotension and ≥3 base deficit;
Retrospective analysis of relatively small (n = 209) population;
No standardized fluid resuscitation scheme employed;
Impact of alcohol and hypoxia unclear;
No gold standard for proof of adequacy of resuscitation.

CHAPTER 9

The Ratio of Blood Products Transfused Affects Mortality in Patients Receiving Massive Transfusions at a Combat Support Hospital

Borgman MA, Spinella PC, Perkins JG, Grathwohl KW, Repine T, Beekley AC, Sebesta J, Jenkins D, Wade CE, Holcomb JB. J Trauma 63(4):805–813, 2007

Abstract   The paper by Borgman et al. was a landmark achievement that led to rapid change in the approach to resuscitation of trauma patients sustaining severe injury with associated blood loss.[1] While there had been much discussion of the importance of higher ratio blood product administration prior to its publication, this paper was the first to clearly demonstrate that mortality was significantly decreased with an increased FFP:RBC ratio in a large number of massively transfused trauma patients. Previous literature had reported similar findings but remained only small in scale and weight. While these anecdotal reports, in conjunction with the observed mortality that accompanied acute coagulopathy, led some to change their practice guidelines and transfusion practices, they did not lead to universal acceptance.

Background   Patients with severe traumatic injuries often present with coagulopathy and require massive transfusion. The risk of death from hemorrhagic shock increases in this population. To treat the coagulopathy of trauma, some have suggested early, aggressive correction using a 1:1 ratio of plasma to red blood cell (RBC) units.

Methods   We performed a retrospective chart review of 246 patients at a US Army combat support hospital, each of who received a massive transfusion ($\geq$10 units of RBCs in 24 hours). Three groups of patients were constructed according to the plasma to RBC ratio transfused during massive transfusion. Mortality rates and the cause of death were compared among groups.

Results   For the low ratio group, the plasma to RBC median ratio was 1:8 (interquartile range, 0:12–1:5), for the medium ratio group, 1:2.5 (interquartile range, 1:3.0–1:2.3), and for the high ratio group, 1:1.4 (interquartile range, 1:1.7–1:1.2) (p < 0.001). Median Injury Severity Score (ISS) was 18 for all groups (interquartile range, 14–25). For low, medium, and high plasma to RBC ratios, overall mortality rates were 65%, 34%, and 19%, (p < 0.001);

and hemorrhage mortality rates were 92.5%, 78%, and 37%, respectively, (p < 0.001). Upon logistic regression, plasma to RBC ratio was independently associated with survival (odds ratio 8.6, 95% confidence interval 2.1–35.2).

Conclusions   In patients with combat-related trauma requiring massive transfusion, a high 1:1.4 plasma to RBC ratio is independently associated with improved survival to hospital discharge, primarily by decreasing death from hemorrhage. For practical purposes, massive transfusion protocols should utilize a 1:1 ratio of plasma to RBCs for all patients who are hypocoagulable with traumatic injuries.

Author Commentary by John B. Holcomb

Our work was the culmination of a decade of near continuous investigation of optimal resuscitation fluids. Building on the recognition that excessive crystalloid was harmful, many authors started investigating blood products using methodology previously reserved for crystalloids. Soon, single and multicenter efforts from the battlefield, in North America, and in Europe all coalesced around the idea that balanced blood product resuscitation was optimal.

The important single center, retrospective effort by Borgman et al. in 2007 described 246 military casualties with massive transfusion. This important work laid the basis for all the later efforts. Three large multicenter civilian studies followed; first a retrospective study in 466 massively transfused civilian patients, then the prospective observational PROMMTT study of 1,245 patients, and finally the prospective and randomized PROPPR study. PROPPR, (n = 680) did not show significant differences in 24-hour or 30-day survival; however, fewer patients exsanguinated in the 1:1:1 group, compared to 1:1:2. No safety issues were identified, despite increased plasma and platelets in the 1:1:1 group. Subsequent analysis revealed that death was significantly decreased at 3 hours, near the median time to hemorrhagic death. In 2017, Cannon et al. published a clinical guideline stating that a balanced transfusion approach is the standard of care for bleeding trauma patients.

Among many others, these four studies have helped change transfusion practice over the last decade. In the early 2000s, it was common to transfuse patients' RBCs and saline with little, if any, plasma or platelets. Ten to twenty liters of saline was frequently infused. A decade later, balanced transfusion of plasma, platelets, and RBCs, and limited crystalloid is the norm. This approach has decreased iatrogenic resuscitation injury, while increasing survival.

What does the future hold for resuscitation? I think that whole blood is the optimal resuscitation fluid for bleeding patients. An entire generation of clinicians have now transfused >10,300 units of whole blood in the deployed military setting with excellent results. A decade ago suggesting that civilian trauma patients be resuscitated with whole blood was often met with quiet laughter. Today, it is a reality in multiple civilian trauma centers and spreading. Starting with dried plasma prehospital and following with cold-stored whole blood seems like the optimal approach, balancing logistics and biologic effect. Interestingly, this was exactly the approach that the Allies used in the last years of World War II. I think they knew what they were doing.

Prehospital resuscitation with blood products (dried and reconstituted near the point of injury) will allow the concepts, proven in the 16 years of war, to expand to the millions of civilians injured every year. In some countries, this idea is already a reality.

Finally, it is extremely important that the Department of Defense (DoD) and National Institutes of Health (NIH) continue to fund clinical resuscitation studies. The progression from single center retrospective through randomized multicenter studies requires enormous effort from literally hundreds of clinicians and substantial funding. The improvement in patient outcomes would not have happened without the funding from those two agencies. It is imperative that they continue their collaborative efforts, so that clinicians can continue to make data driven improvements in resuscitation science.

Expert Commentary by Parker J. Hu and Jeffrey D. Kerby

Historically, transfusion strategies mimicked those seen in the elective surgical and medical population, with blood products administered in response to laboratory derangements. Treatment of coagulopathy was typically delayed and inadequate, resulting in continued bleeding and patient death. Given the low incidence of hemorrhagic shock requiring massive transfusion at civilian trauma centers, large trials were lacking. This study was a retrospective analysis of trauma patients admitted to a combat support hospital in Iraq over a nearly 2-year period. Patients requiring massive transfusion (>10 units within 24 hours of arrival) were stratified into three cohorts of increasing FFP:RBC ratio. The decrease in absolute mortality from 65% in the low ratio group to 19% in the high ratio group, as well as the decrease in mortality on multivariate analysis, was profound. Concurrent to these findings was the increased availability and use of thawed plasma at most major trauma centers that facilitated increased ratios of FFP:RBC during the early phases of resuscitation. Of interest, a subsequent paper supported the concept that the survival benefit associated with MTPs was likely due to early and aggressive use of plasma and blood products unrelated to changes in product ratio.[2]

Aside from the obvious limitation of this being a retrospective analysis, the authors did note the potential that patients receiving lower FFP:RBC ratios may have done so as a function of dying prior to having the ability to receive plasma. This concern was later correctly defined in a subsequent paper as survival bias.[3] As ratios are not fixed over time, application of a time-varying covariate to FFP:RBC ratios questioned the results of the Borgman paper, while acknowledging the clear rationale for higher FFP:RBC ratios. Subsequent prospective, randomized trials addressed survival bias along with other limitations of previous studies.[4] While the PROPPR trial was underpowered to show a 24-hour or 30-day mortality benefit for higher FFP:Platelet:RBC ratios, the study did show higher rates of hemostasis and less mortality from hemorrhage at 24 hours in the high ratio cohort.

In conclusion, the study published by Borgman et al. was transformative and informed further investigation into the benefits of high ratio blood product transfusion. This analysis, along with availability of thawed plasma, were catalysts for a change in practice that has become a staple of modern-day resuscitation strategies.

REFERENCES

1. Borgman MA, Spinella PC, Perkins JG, et al. The ratio of blood products transfused affects mortality in patients receiving massive transfusions at a combat support hospital. *J Trauma*. 2007; 63: 805–813.
2. Riskin DJ, Tsai TC, Riskin L, et al. Massive transfusion protocols: The role of aggressive resuscitation versus product ratio in mortality reduction. *J Am Coll Surg*. 2009; 209: 198–205.
3. Snyder CW, Weinberg JA, McGwin G, et al. The relationship of blood product ratio to mortality: Survival benefit or survival bias? *J Trauma*. 2009; 66: 358–364.
4. Holcomb JB, Tilley BC, Baraniuk S, et al. Transfusion of plasma, platelets, and red blood cells in a 1:1:1 vs a 1:1:2 ratio and mortality in patients with severe trauma: The PROPPR randomized clinical trial. *JAMA*. 2015; 313: 471–482.

Editor Notes: This was a retrospective review of military wounded who underwent "massive transfusion," which focused on survival related to the ratio of packed red cells to plasma. A 1:1 ratio was found to be associated with the lowest mortality and was highly predictive of survival (OR 8.9) in their multivariate analysis. As a result of this and subsequent investigations, clinicians altered the way that institutions approach the massively bleeding patient: massive transfusion protocols were devised; blood products were made immediately available; and crystalloid infusions were minimized. While the study had numerous potential limitations, it focused our attention on this critical aspect of resuscitation and ultimately led to improvements in patient survival.

Limitations:

Population was confined to young healthy soldiers with severe penetrating war wounds;
Massive transfusion was defined as 10 units/24 hours;
Potential survival bias.

CHAPTER 10

Hypothermia in Trauma Victims: An Ominous Predictor of Survival

Jurkovich GJ, Greiser WB, Luterman A, Curreri PW.
J Trauma 27(9):1019–1024, 1987

Abstract Hypothermia in trauma patients is generally considered an ominous sign, although the actual temperature at which hypothermia affects survival is ill defined. In this study, the impact of body core hypothermia on outcome in 71 adult trauma patients with Injury Severity Scores (ISS) greater than or equal to 25 was analyzed. Forty-two percent of the patients had a core temperature (Tc) below 34°C, 23% below 33°C, and 13% below 32°C. The mortality of hypothermia patients was consistently greater than those who remained warm, regardless of index core temperature. Mortality if Tc was less than 34°C = 40%, less than 33°C = 69%, less than 32°C = 100%, whereas mortality if Tc was greater than or equal to 34°C = 7%, and greater than or equal to 32°C = 10%. Mortality and the incidence of hypothermia increased with higher ISS, massive fluid resuscitation, and the presence of shock. Within each subgroup (i.e., greater ISS, massive fluid administration, shock) the mortality of hypothermic patients was significantly higher than those who remained warm. No patient whose core temperature fell below 32°C survived.

Author Commentary by Gregory J. Jurkovich

Following the Vietnam War and the return of military surgeons to civilian practices, the county hospitals of the United States became the *de facto* trauma centers, bringing home learned lessons in surgical care. These urban "safety-net" centers were the training ground of a generation of surgeons in the care of the injured patient, initially from penetrating wounds of urban violence, but with time, the blunt trauma patients from motor vehicle crashes, falls, industrial injuries, and the like. While trauma remained a, generally, "neglected disease" in terms of research dollars and public funding for infrastructure,[1,2] the American College of Surgeons Committee on Trauma was working hard to define the essential elements of a trauma center, creating the verification review program in 1987.[3,4] The concept of temperature control or prevention of hypothermia in the injured patient was not one of the considerations of the essential elements of trauma center verification, nor was it part of the ABCs of the early Advanced Trauma Life Support (ATLS®) courses. Indeed, with the development of cardiac surgery and the essential role of cardioplegia while "on pump," and the need for hypothermia to preserve organs prior to transplantations, hypothermia was not considered harmful; it was an expected part of injury and elective operations and was generally thought to be an advantageous response to injury.[5]

It was within this context that the above paper was presented at the 1986 Annual Meeting of the American Association for the Surgery of Trauma, alongside a similar article by Luna and colleagues.[6] Both acknowledged that hypothermia was a well-recognized consequence of severe injury, and both documented its incidence and associated factors. The paper by Jurkovich et al. made the additional observation that correlated the degree of hypothermia with mortality, making the bold statement that below 32°C survival would not occur, and believing this to be independent of injury severity. Namely, hypothermia itself adversely influenced mortality and was not simply a response to the severity of the injury. In this retrospective review of 71 patients, all patients had an ISS > 25, and all were direct scene ground transports. The article examined patients based on injury severity categories, presence of hypotensive shock, fluid administration, age, and operative interventions. Mortality was uniformly 100% for those with a core body temperature of 32°C or colder.

These papers begged the question of whether it was the hypothermia per se or the severity of the injury producing the hypothermia that was responsible for the mortality. As such, they fostered numerous subsequent articles and experiments looking at the role of rewarming, and eventually, at preventing hypothermia from ever occurring in trauma patients. This spawned the widespread use of Level 1® rewarmer, Bair Huggers®, and other warming devices in the ED and OR for all cases. A subsequent sentinel work by Gentilello et al. demonstrated in a prospective, randomized clinical trial that rapid reversal of hypothermia was lifesaving.[7] The overriding hypothesis remains that hypothermia in the polytrauma patient increases capillary permeability, fluid requirements, energy expenditure, and perhaps most importantly, a coagulopathy that cannot be corrected with blood product administration.[8]

With this recognition and incorporation of hypothermia prevention strategies in all aspect of trauma care, from the field to the OR, the occurrence of hypothermia to 32°C has largely been eliminated. Indeed, it is the rare patient that needs active rewarming in the trauma ICU. The ATLS® course has adopted "environmental control" as part of the "E" of the ABCs of the primary survey, and hypothermia prevention devises are now required equipment for all ACS COT verified trauma centers.

REFERENCES

1. *Accidental Death and Disability: The Neglected Disease of Modern Society*. Washington, DC, 1966.
2. Gaston SR. Accidental death and disability: The neglected disease of modern society: A progress report. *J Trauma*. 1971; 11(3): 195–206.
3. American College of Surgeons, Committee on Trauma. *Resources for Optimal Care of the Injured Patient*. Chicago, IL: American College of Surgeons, Committee on Trauma; 1990. iii, 79 p.
4. ACS COT. ACS COT Verifcation Reveiw Consultation 2017. Available from: https://www .facs.org/quality-programs/trauma/vrc/about.
5. Goldberg MJ, Roe CF. Temperature changes during anesthesia and operations. *Arch Surg*. 1966; 93(2): 365–369.
6. Luna GK, Maier RV, Pavlin EG, Anardi D, Copass MK, Oreskovich MR. Incidence and effect of hypothermia in seriously injured patients. *J Trauma*. 1987; 27(9): 1014–1018.
7. Gentilello LM, Jurkovich GJ, Stark MS, Hassantash SA, O'Keefe GE. Is hypothermia in the victim of major trauma protective or harmful? A randomized, prospective study. *Ann Surg*. 1997; 226(4): 439–447; discussion 447–449.
8. Gubler KD, Gentilello LM, Hassantash SA, Maier RV. The impact of hypothermia on dilutional coagulopathy. *J Trauma*. 1994; 36(6): 847–851.

Expert Commentary by Hasan B. Alam

"Double-edged sword"—Something that has or can have both favorable and unfavorable consequences.

Merriam-Webster Dictionary

The impact of this paper, which was published three decades ago, is difficult to imagine now, but it has clearly influenced the thinking of a whole generation of trauma surgeons. Dr. Jurkovich reviewed the charts of 71 severely injured trauma victims in Alabama (not a cold place) and discovered that mortality of hypothermic patients was significantly higher than those who stayed warm. Mortality and incidence of hypothermia increased with higher injury severity scores, resuscitation volumes, and shock. He reported a stepwise increase in mortality as the core body temperature dropped, with no survivors below core temperature of 32°C. These findings were novel and controversial at that time. The discussion section accompanying the paper captures the question-answer session at the meeting. Nearly every prominent trauma surgeon who got up to comment on this paper, expressed their bias in favor of hypothermia as a cytoprotective modality. In fact, many described experiences with otherwise non-salvageable patients who survived just because they were hypothermic. This love for hypothermia was not surprising considering that time period. In the late 1980s, we had accumulated decades of experience with hypothermia, and therapeutic cooling was firmly established in the thriving fields of cardiac surgery, organ transplant, and complex neurosurgery. This paper challenged the dogma and pointed out that cold trauma patients die at an alarmingly high rate. Although a small retrospective study, this paper progressively gained more attention and changed how trauma surgeons viewed hypothermia. It also led to many other developments. For example, if hypothermia was bad, then active rewarming should logically be beneficial. Aggressive rewarming protocols were developed and implemented,[1] and indeed patients that failed to respond to rewarming protocols were noted to have excessively high mortality.[2]

So, how do we reconcile the well-established protective properties of hypothermia in non-trauma patients against the high mortality rates in the hypothermic trauma population? Is this a cause and effect relationship or just an epiphenomenon? Although no randomized clinical trials have been conducted to test the therapeutic benefits of hypothermia in trauma patients, numerous well-designed pre-clinical studies clearly support this concept.[3] It should be emphasized up front that *induced hypothermia* and *hypothermia secondary to shock* are very different entities.[4,5] Induced hypothermia is therapeutic in nature, whereas hypothermia, seen in severely traumatized patients, is a sign of tissue ischemia and failure of homeostatic mechanisms to maintain normal body temperature. It is clear from the literature that rapid induction of deep/profound hypothermia ($<15°C$) can improve an otherwise dismal outcome after exsanguinating cardiac arrest.[3-5] Depending on the degree of hypothermia, good outcomes have been achieved with cardiac arrests of 15, 20, 30, and even 90 minutes in canine models. Furthermore, the period of hypothermia can be safely extended to 180 minutes if blood is replaced with organ preservation fluids and low flow cardiopulmonary bypass is maintained during this period. Large animal experiments provide convincing evidence that lethal vascular injuries, along with solid organ and bowel injuries can be repaired under profound hypothermic protection with excellent long-term survival and low complication rates. To achieve the best results, hypothermia must be induced rapidly ($2°C$/minute) and reversed at a slower rate ($0.5°C$/minute). Hypothermia not only modulates metabolism, but also influences a wide variety of cellular and sub-cellular mechanisms that can be beneficial long after the period of hypothermia, such as alteration in transcription of numerous genes. Since the publication of this landmark paper by Jurkovich, an extensive body of literature has accumulated that suggests that hypothermia is indeed a double-edged sword. The biological processes in mammals are designed to work optimally at a certain temperature, and deviation from this temperature can have adverse consequences.[4] We also know that maintaining normal body temperature is an energy dependent process and patients that are in severe shock progressively become hypothermic, which is an ominous sign. However, active and careful induction of hypothermia for a limited period is clearly different, and it can allow us to preserve key organs during repair of otherwise lethal injuries.[5] The way I look at it, "All dead patients are cold but not all cold patients are dead." In fact, the data are compelling enough that the FDA has approved a clinical trial (ClinicalTrials.gov Identifier:NCT01042015), and a prospective clinical trial is underway to test the feasibility of inducing profound hypothermia as a lifesaving strategy in patients with lethal but potentially fixable injuries.[6]

Like most things in medicine, the pendulum keeps on swinging. This is especially true for critical care therapies, where treatments that were once loved, were abandoned for a period, only to be embraced yet again. Hypothermia is not by itself all good or bad—it depends upon whether we are looking at it as a marker of shock or as a therapeutic tool.

REFERENCES

1. Gentilello LM, Cobean RA, Offner PJ, Soderberg RW, Jurkovich GJ. Continuous arterio-venous rewarming: Rapid reversal of hypothermia in critically ill patients. *J Trauma*. 1992; 32(3): 316–325; discussion 325–327.
2. Gentilello LM, Jurkovich GJ, Stark MS, Hassantash SA, O'Keefe GE. Is hypothermia in the victim of major trauma protective or harmful? A randomized, prospective study. *Ann Surg*. 1997; 226(4): 439–447; discussion 447–449.
3. Alam HB, Pusateri AE, Kindzelski A, et al. HYPOSTAT workshop participants: Hypothermia and hemostasis in severe trauma—A new crossroads workshop report. *J Trauma Acute Care Surg*. 2012; 73(4): 809–817. doi:10.1097/TA.0b013e318265d1b8.
4. Finkelstein RA, Alam HB. Induced hypothermia for trauma: Current research and practice. *J Intensive Care Med*. 2010; 25(4): 205–226. doi:10.1177/0885066610366919.
5. Alam HB. Translational barriers and opportunities for emergency preservation and resuscitation in severe injuries. *Br J Surg*. 2012; 99(Suppl 1): 29–39. doi:10.1002/bjs.7756.
6. Tisherman SA, Alam HB, Rhee PM, Scalea TM, Drabek T, Forsythe RM, Kochanek PM. Development of the emergency preservation and resuscitation for cardiac arrest from trauma clinical trial. *J Trauma Acute Care Surg*. 2017; 83(5): 803809. doi:10.1097/TA.0000000000001585.

Editor Notes: The authors evaluated 71 patients with severe truncal trauma (ISS $\geq$ 25) and demonstrated an increase in mortality when core temperature decreased below 34°C. They also noted that >5 liters of crystalloid and >5 units of blood were associated with a higher likelihood of hypothermia and subsequent increased mortality.

Limitations:

Retrospective study;
Limited size young adult, mostly penetrating (70%) patient population;
Only severely injured patients analyzed;
Consistency of rewarming techniques unclear.

CHAPTER 11

Defining the Limits of Resuscitative Emergency Department Thoracotomy: A Contemporary Western Trauma Association Perspective

Moore EE, Knudson MM, Burlew CC, Inaba K, Dicker RA, Biffl WL, Malhotra AK, Schreiber MA, Browder TD, Coimbra R, Gonzalez EA, Meredith JW, Livingston DH, Kaups KL., WTA Study Group. J Trauma 70(2):334–339, 2011

Abstract   This paper reports a multiyear, multiple institution study conducted by a distinguished group of investigators. It attempts to supply data that could serve as a basis for evidence-based guidelines governing the use of EDT in trauma patients. It reports a prospective collection of observations regarding 56 successful applications of emergency department thoracotomy (EDT) occurring over 6 years in 18 trauma centers (i.e., 108 institution-years). This amounts to about one survivor per trauma center *every 2 years*. The actual number of EDTs performed by the reporting institutions is not reported, nor is anything indicated about the physiologic state, operative selection criteria, or anatomic injuries of the nonsurvivors. These latter data were regarded by the investigators as "nonessential" to the intention of the study.

Background   Since the promulgation of emergency department (ED) thoracotomy over 40 years ago, there has been an ongoing search to define when this heroic resuscitative effort is futile. In this era of health care reform, the generation of accurate data is imperative for developing patient care guidelines. The purpose of this prospective multicenter study was to identify injury patterns and physiologic profiles at ED arrival that are compatible with survival.

Methods   Eighteen institutions representing the Western Trauma Association commenced enrollment in January 2003; data were collected prospectively.

Results   During the ensuing 6 years, 56 patients survived to hospital discharge. Mean age was 31.3 years (15–64 years), and 93% were male. As expected, survival was predominant in those with thoracic injuries (77%), followed by abdomen (9%), extremity (7%), neck (4%), and head (4%). The most common injury was a ventricular stab wound (30%), followed by a gunshot wound to the lung (16%); 9% of survivors sustained blunt trauma, 34% underwent prehospital cardiopulmonary resuscitation (CPR), and the presenting base deficit was >25 mequiv/L in 18%. Relevant to futile care, there were survivors of blunt torso injuries with CPR up to 9 minutes and penetrating torso wounds up to 15 minutes. Asystole was documented at ED arrival in seven patients (12%); all these patients had pericardial tamponade, and three (43%) had good functional neurologic recovery at hospital discharge.

Conclusions   Resuscitative thoracotomy in the ED can be considered futile care when (a) prehospital CPR exceeds 10 minutes after blunt trauma without a response, (b) prehospital CPR exceeds 15 minutes after penetrating trauma without a response, and (c) asystole is the presenting rhythm and there is no pericardial tamponade.

Author Commentary by Ernest E. Moore

Emergency department thoracotomy (EDT) for resuscitation of the moribund patient with penetrating cardiovascular wounds was introduced by the Ben Taub Hospital in 1967. EDT was adopted widely with unbridled enthusiasm. Dr. Ben Eiseman hired me in 1976 to establish a trauma center at the Denver General Hospital (DGH). DGH was a prototypic county hospital, located in the impoverished section where much of the inner-city violence occurred. At the first Morbidity and Mortality conference I attended, a patient was presented for death following an EDT, and Dr. Eiseman astutely noted there were no published criteria addressing indications for this "high intensity/low yield heroic procedure." Thus, as the Chief of Trauma, my first assignment was to define these criteria. We were well positioned to study this topic, because all injured patients in Denver County were delivered to the DGH by the Denver EMS that was housed within the hospital. Thus, prehospital details were readily available and could be confirmed by direct communication with the paramedic involved. We began a prospective database, which continues today, over 40 years later. Our first efforts at defining indications/limitations of EDT were published in 1979, and we subsequently have published refinements of criteria as our experience expanded. We acknowledged that documented asystole at the scene was a marker of futility, but our urban EMS transport system, like many in the United States, did not routinely monitor cardiac activity in the field. Consequently, we focused on duration of prehospital CPR and status of the patient at arrival in the ED to determine when EDT would represent futile care. Remarkably consistent was the maximal duration of prehospital CPR for survival was 15 minutes for penetrating wounds and 10 minutes for blunt trauma. We documented survival in patients arriving asystolic with pericardial tamponade. But our results were challenged with the understandable reservation that they represented a single institution with a rigorous protocol for EDT. Therefore, we suggested a multicenter trial through the Western Trauma Association (WTA) to determine the applicability of our long-standing recommendations.

The results of the WTA prospective observational trial validated the Denver criteria, as summarized in the abstract. Of note, a third of the patients who survived EDT had ongoing prehospital CPR, a condition some guidelines consider unsalvageable. Furthermore, patients survived prehospital CPR following blunt trauma. Finally, patients with asystole as well as PEA survived rendering the utility of ED ultrasound limited for this purpose. While the data from the WTA trial provide assurance that CPR >10 minutes for blunt trauma and >15 minutes for penetration wounds are reasonable indications to forgo EDT, there are reports of survival exceeding these times. A conspicuous limitation of this study is the inability to ascertain when CPR is required; that is, CPR may be initiated prematurely providing misleading information. But until we have point of care availability of metabolic markers of nonsurvival in the field, duration of CPR stratified by injury mechanism may be the best we have at the moment.

Expert Commentary by Robert F. Buckman

The authors report no actionable conclusions. This failure after such a big effort reflects the complexities of the issue particularly: (1) the innumerable variables involved in the causes, degrees and hemodynamic trajectories of cardiovascular compromise associated with trauma; (2) the fact that open chest resuscitation is usually just one element of a maximum resuscitation effort; and (3) the fact that the procedures, including pericardiotomy, cardiac injury repair, aortic clamping, hilar clamping, cardiac massage, and others, performed during the course of an EDT vary according to the anatomic injuries and the physiologic condition of the patient. A further difficulty with the reliability of the data is the possible modification of fluid resuscitation practices, including the implementation of so-called Damage Control Resuscitation, over the period of the study.

The data indicate that, within the experience of the reporting institutions, there were no survivors in the following circumstances:

- Prehospital CPR greater than 10 minutes after blunt trauma *without response*
- Prehospital CPR greater than 15 minutes after penetrating injury *without response*
- Asystole is the presenting rhythm and there is *no pericardial tamponade*

The data appear to provide evidence-based guidelines, but they do not. There were only 56 survivors reported, and each of the research findings incorporates a significant qualification.

- The prehospital CPR times for penetrating and blunt trauma patients, beyond which there were no survivors, had the qualification that the patient had no *response* during CPR, but the definition of a *response* is not given.
- The qualification regarding patients with asystole is that the patient had no pericardial tamponade, but there is no indication of whether the presence or absence of tamponade was known from preoperative ultrasound or from operative observation of the pericardium.

In summary, the finding of the paper is that EDT was unsuccessful in the hands of the reporting institutions when undertaken for patients outside stipulated physiological and circumstantial characteristics. It is *not* concluded that EDT must always be futile in cases outside these limits, or that reliable guidelines could be based on these findings. In fact, the authors acknowledge that their observations regarding the "limits" of EDT, suggested in the title of this paper, are contradicted by several other reports in the published literature.

Editor Notes: Multiple trauma centers prospectively collected data on emergency room thoracotomy to better understand the limits of resuscitation, or "futility," in this patient population. The use of resuscitative thoracotomy was recommended only when prehospital CPR was less than 10 minutes in blunt trauma, or less than 15 minutes in penetrating trauma.

Limitations:

Prospective observational study;
Limited data revealed;
Possible variability in quality of resuscitative intervention;
Does not take into consideration the possibility of organ donation.

CHAPTER 12

Resuscitative Endovascular Balloon Occlusion of the Aorta (REBOA) as an Adjunct for Hemorrhagic Shock

Stannard A, Eliason JE, Rasmussen TE. J Trauma 71(6):1869–1872, 2011

Abstract   Understanding the potential for this paper to be a landmark reference, and because it was aimed at opening the aperture of endovascular skills to other disciplines (i.e., to the general and trauma surgery communities), it was written deliberately as a procedure note. The paper outlines five steps in the performance of REBOA as well as the materials available at that time needed for each step. Out of caution, the manuscript also listed considerations and potential hazards of each of the steps in this procedure. Notably, although more agile REBOA technologies are now available, the zones, the steps, and the potential hazards outlined in this original manuscript are still relevant for those establishing standard procedures for the performance of this resuscitative maneuver.[1,2]

Author Commentary by Todd E. Rasmussen

The 2011 manuscript "Resuscitative Endovascular Balloon Occlusion of the Aorta (REBOA) as an Adjunct for Hemorrhagic Shock" was submitted at the prompting of then Editor-in-Chief of the *Journal of Trauma*, Dr. Basil A. Pruitt, who recognized the changing landscape of hemorrhage control and resuscitation and the growing role of endovascular techniques in this space. At the time, two epidemiologic studies had been performed by the US military identifying the lethality of non-compressible torso hemorrhage and a third, the Eastridge "Death on the Battlefield" project, was underway.[3–5] The military had initiated a research program to assess resuscitative endovascular balloon occlusion of the aorta as an alternative to direct aortic clamping via laparotomy or thoracotomy. By 2011, initial porcine models had shown the endovascular approach held promise and a new device was in the early prototype stage.[6–8] The inability of traditional, open surgical approaches to reduce mortality from this injury scenario also created an urgency for a new approach, one that could be rendered more effectively as a stabilizing maneuver and earlier in the course of hemorrhagic shock.

Although the publication christened the term REBOA and defined the aortic occlusion zones, the maneuver itself was hardly new. In 1954, then Major Carl Hughes published a case series from the Korean War in which a rudimentary endovascular balloon device was inflated inside of the aorta as an intraoperative rescue maneuver and several case series, still using antiquated technologies, appeared in publication in the 1980s and 1990s.[9–11] It wasn't until after the revolution of endovascular technologies had occurred between 1990 and 2010 that REBOA could be legitimately reappraised for its potential to shift the management of bleeding and shock. Remember, at the time, the seemingly immovable mortality from ruptured abdominal aortic aneurysms was, for the first time in five decades, being positively affected by the use of endovascular approaches, including REBOA. There was a sense, an enthusiasm, and a plausible clinical model showing that REBOA would work in severely injured and shocked patients.

By some counts, the manuscript has been cited nearly 1,000 times, and its appeal is a testament to the vision of Dr. Pruitt as he encouraged the paper for the *Journal of Trauma* during his final months as Editor-in-Chief. As an indication to interest in the paper, and as one can read in the publication fine print, the paper was submitted to the journal on October 31, 2011; it was accepted the next day, on November 1, and it was published the following month, in December 2011. While the role of endovascular balloon occlusion of the aorta in the management of bleeding and shock was not yet fully determined, this publication occurred at a unique juncture in time and will always be recognized as the REBOA paper. It's my hope that the manuscript continues to have enduring value and that it will serve as a guide for those considering this and other endovascular approaches in the management of the severely injured or ill patient.

REFERENCES

1. Rasmussen TE, Eliason JL. Military-civilian partnership in device innovation: Development, commercialization and application of Resuscitative Endovascular Balloon Occlusion of the Aorta (REBOA). *J Trauma Acute Care Surg.* 2017; 83(4): 732–735. doi:10.1097/TA.0000000000001661.
2. Rasmussen TE, Franklin CJ, Eliason JL. Surgical Innovation: Resuscitative endovascular balloon occlusion of the aorta for hemorrhagic shock. *JAMA Surg.* 2017; 152(11): 1072–1073.
3. Holcomb JB, McMullin NR, Pearse L, Caruso J, Wade CE, Oetjen-Gerdes L, Champion HR, et al. Causes of death in U.S. Special Operations Forces in the global war on terrorism 2001–2004. *Ann Surg.* 2007; 986–991.
4. Kelly JF, Ritenour AE, McLaughlin DF, Bagg KA, Apodaca AN, Mallak CT, Pearse L, et al. Injury severity and causes of death from Operation Iraqi Freedom and Operation Enduring Freedom: 2003–2004 versus 2006. *J Trauma.* 2008; 64(2 Suppl): S21–S26; discussion S26–S27.
5. Eastridge BJ, Mabry RL, Seguin P, Cantrell J, Tops T, Uribe P, Mallett O, Zubko T, Oetjen-Gerdes L, Rasmussen TE, et al. Death on the battlefield (2001–2011): Implications for the future of combat casualty care. *J Trauma Acute Care Surg.* 2012; 73: S431–S437.
6. Eliason JL, Rasmussen TE. US Patent 9,131,874, 2015. Fluoroscopy-independent, endovascular aortic occlusion system.

7. White JM, Cannon JW, Stannard A, Markov NP, Spencer JR, Rasmussen TE. Endovascular balloon occlusion of the aorta is superior to resuscitative thoracotomy with aortic clamping in a porcine model of hemorrhagic shock. *Surgery*. 2011; 150: 400–409.
8. Scott DJ, Eliason JL, Villamaria C, Morrison JJ, Houston R, Spencer JR, Rasmussen TE. A novel fluoroscopy-free, resuscitative endovascular aortic balloon occlusion system in a model of hemorrhagic shock. *J Trauma Acute Care Surg*. 2013; 75: 122–128.
9. Hughes CW. Use of an intra-aortic balloon catheter tamponade for controlling intraabdominal hemorrhage in man. *Surgery*. 1954; 36: 65–68.
10. Gupta BK, Khaneja SC, Flores L, Eastlick L, Longmore W, Shaftan GW. The role of intra-aortic balloon occlusion in penetrating abdominal trauma. *J Trauma*. 1989; 29: 861–865.
11. Low RB, Longmore W, Rubinstein R, Flores L, Wolvek S. Preliminary report on the use of the Percluder occluding aortic balloon in human beings. *Ann Emerg Med*. 1986; 15: 1466–1469.

Expert Commentary by James N. Bogert

Occlusion of the aorta for select patients in hemorrhagic shock has been a part of the trauma surgeons' armamentarium for decades.[1] Both open and endovascular strategies for aortic occlusion were described as far back as the 1950s.[2] However, for a variety of reasons including poor results and cumbersome equipment, the endovascular approach fell out of the general and trauma surgeons' consciousness for most of the last century. In the 1990s and early 2000s, when endovascular techniques revolutionized the treatment of ruptured abdominal aortic aneurysms, endovascular strategies for hemorrhage began to reenter the minds of trauma surgeons.[3] However, with poor exposure to these techniques in training, the pathway to disseminating this technique in the trauma world was unclear: Resuscitative Endovascular Balloon Occlusion of the Aorta (REBOA) remained an interesting, yet relatively obscure topic.

The publication of "Resuscitative Endovascular Balloon Occlusion of the Aorta (REBOA) as an Adjunct for Hemorrhagic Shock" marks an inflection point in the story of REBOA. Before this publication, REBOA was an interesting oddity that seemed feasible in highly specialized centers with a very specific set of capabilities. After this publication, REBOA seemed more accessible to the "ordinary" level I trauma center. The step-by-step description of the REBOA procedure and its many associated pitfalls and technical tips were integrated into early military courses, such as Endovascular Skills for Trauma and Resuscitation (ESTAR), and remains highly pertinent in today's American College of Surgeons' Basic Endovascular Skills for Trauma (BEST) course.[4,5] The number of centers capable of REBOA has expanded dramatically thanks to the training available through these courses and drawing on the lessons from this publication.

With the acute care surgery community embracing this new endovascular era, the multi-institution AORTA registry has been established to monitor outcomes from this new procedure with early results showing REBOA to be comparable to resuscitative thoracotomy.[6] As more acute care surgeons, who are present in the hospital 24/7, gain the skill set to insert a REBOA, the application to non-traumatic hemorrhage is showing promise. Acute care surgeons have placed REBOA for, among other indications, post-partum hemorrhage and gastrointestinal bleeding with good success.[7,8]

As REBOA use has expanded, our awareness of its associated complications has improved.[9] While newer devices and improved technology make the procedure less complex, the endovascular principles described in this publication remain the cornerstone to safe REBOA insertion by a growing number of acute care surgeons today. The coming years will yield further improvements and implementation of REBOA into practice. At the core of this expanded availability of endovascular techniques for hemorrhage control will be the techniques and principles described in "Resuscitative Endovascular Balloon Occlusion of the Aorta (REBOA) as an Adjunct for Hemorrhagic Shock."

REFERENCES

1. Ledgerwood AM, Kazmers M, Lucas CE. The role of thoracic aortic occlusion for massive hemoperitoneum. *J Trauma*. 1976; 16(8): 610–615.
2. Hughes CW. Use of an intra-aortic balloon catheter tamponade for controlling intra-abdominal hemorrhage in man. *Surgery*. 1954; 36(1): 65–68.
3. Matsuoka S, Uchiyama K, Shima H, Ohishi S, Nojiri Y, Ogata H. Temporary percutaneous aortic balloon occlusion to enhance fluid resuscitation prior to definitive embolization of posttraumatic liver hemorrhage. *Cardiovasc Intervent Radiol*. 2001; 24(4): 274–276.
4. Villamaria CY, Eliason JL, Napolitano LM, Stansfield RB, Spencer JR, Rasmussen TE. Endovascular Skills for Trauma and Resuscitative Surgery (ESTARS) course: Curriculum development, content validation, and program assessment. *J Trauma Acute Care Surg*. 2014; 76(4): 929–935; discussion 35–36.
5. Brenner M, Hoehn M, Pasley J, Dubose J, Stein D, Scalea T. Basic endovascular skills for trauma course: Bridging the gap between endovascular techniques and the acute care surgeon. *J Trauma Acute Care Surg*. 2014; 77(2): 286–291.
6. DuBose JJ, Scalea TM, Brenner M, Skiada D, Inaba K, Cannon J, et al. The AAST prospective Aortic Occlusion for Resuscitation in Trauma and Acute Care Surgery (AORTA) registry: Data on contemporary utilization and outcomes of aortic occlusion and resuscitative balloon occlusion of the aorta (REBOA). *J Trauma Acute Care Surg*. 2016; 81(3): 409–419.
7. Manzano-Nuñez R, Escobar-Vidarte MF, Orlas CP, Herrera-Escobar JP, Galvagno SM, Melendez JJ, et al. Resuscitative endovascular balloon occlusion of the aorta deployed by acute care surgeons in patients with morbidly adherent placenta: A feasible solution for two lives in peril. *World J Emerg Surg*. 2018; 13: 44.
8. Hoehn MR, Hansraj NZ, Pasley AM, Brenner M, Cox SR, Pasley JD, et al. Resuscitative endovascular balloon occlusion of the aorta for non-traumatic intra-abdominal hemorrhage. *Eur J Trauma Emerg Surg*. 2018.
9. Davidson AJ, Russo RM, Reva VA, Brenner ML, Moore LJ, Ball C, et al. The pitfalls of resuscitative endovascular balloon occlusion of the aorta: Risk factors and mitigation strategies. *J Trauma Acute Care Surg*. 2018; 84(1): 192–202.

Editor Notes: This was an important study demonstrating the value of intravascular shunts in wartime. One hundred and twenty-six extremity vascular injuries underwent placement of shunts. No complications were noted, and the patency rates were extremely high. This paper lead to the widespread use of shunts in the care of both combat and civilian trauma victims with vascular injuries.

Limitations:

Small series;
No control group;
Limited follow-up data;
Relationship to amputation unclear (7% had amputation);
Most shunts were < 2-hour duration.

CHAPTER 13

The Clinical Utility of Computed Tomographic Scanning and Neurologic Examination in the Management of Patients with Minor Head Injuries

Shackford SR, Wald SL, Ross SE, Cogbill TH, Hoyt DB, Morris JA,
Mucha PA, Pachter HL, Sugerman HJ, O'Malley K, et al.

J Trauma 33(3):385–394, 1992

Abstract The evaluation and management of patients with minor head injury (MHI: history of loss of consciousness or posttraumatic amnesia and a GCS score greater than 12) remain controversial. Recommendations vary from routine admission without computed tomographic (CT) scanning to mandatory CT scanning and admission to CT scanning without admission for selected patients. Previous reports examining this issue have included patients with associated non-CNS injuries who confound the interpretation of the data and affect outcome. We hypothesized that patients with MHI and no other reason for admission with normal neurologic examinations and normal CT scans would have a negligible risk of neurologic deterioration requiring surgical intervention. To validate this hypothesis, we studied 2,766 patients with an isolated MHI admitted to seven trauma centers between January 1, 1988, and December 31, 1991. There were 1,898 male patients and 868 female patients; injury was blunt in 99%. A neurologic examination and a CT scan were performed on 2,166 patients; 933 patients had normal neurologic examinations and normal CT scans, and none required craniotomy; 1,170 patients had normal CT scans, and none required craniotomy; 2,112 patients had normal neurologic examinations and 59 required a craniotomy. The sensitivity of the CT scan was 100%, with positive predictive value of 10%, negative predictive value of 100%, and specificity of 51%. The use of CT alone as a diagnostic modality would have saved 3,924 hospital days, including 814 ICU days and $1,509,012 in-hospital charges. Based on these data, we believe that CT scanning is essential in the management of patients with MHI, and that if the neurologic examination is normal and the scan is negative, then patients can be safely discharged from the emergency room.

Author Commentary by Steven R. Shackford

By the late 1980s, there was considerable variability in the management of patients with mild head injury (MHI). The available literature consisted of single-center studies of relatively small cohorts and included patients with multiple associated injuries. These studies certainly had internal validity, but there remained a significant knowledge gap not only about external validity, but also concerning an acceptable definition of MHI, as well as the utility of routine CT scanning, the usefulness of the neurologic exam (NEx), and the necessity of routine admission for observation even if the scan and the NEx were negative. Additionally, the inclusion of patients with associated injuries could affect the management in terms of imaging and admission to the hospital. We, therefore, decided to study *isolated* MHI.

The Western Trauma Association Multicenter Trials Group provided a platform and an excellent opportunity to address these knowledge gaps using a multicenter format (comprised of centers with differing approaches to the management of MHI).

The success and the strength of any multicenter design are dependent upon the degree of commitment of each principal investigators (PI), and the willingness of the PI to be free of confirmation bias when submitting data. Commitment was critical as this work was performed with rudimentary computer data capture and analysis (i.e., prior to the introduction of such tools as REDCap).

Each PI participated in the explicit definition of all variables and the methodology for analysis. Because most institutions at this time were looking at cost containment, routine admission for MHI would be costly. Thus, we added a "cost" or "charge" analogue to our analysis. This "charge" analysis was pertinent because it was felt by many that routine CT scanning of MHI was an unnecessary charge because "it was usually normal."

Participating centers ranged in size from 390 beds to 1,300 beds. To account for the trauma center volume, the duration of data entry was varied (1–3 years) so that there was a relatively similar number of patients from each participating institution.

All of the authors enthusiastically embraced the work and were hopeful that it would yield a useful algorithm for the management of MHI.

Expert Commentary by David H. Livingston

At the time of this study, the evaluation and treatment of patients with minimal head injuries occupied enormous resources. Almost all busy trauma services were admitting and discharging a half dozen patients a day who sustained a loss of consciousness and regardless of the findings on imaging, were admitted for "neurologic observation." Some were intoxicated, some were not. Some had an altered mental status, most did not. The increased use of cranial CT scanning in the mid-1980s demonstrated that most of these patients had no intracranial injuries, but some did and some even required craniotomy. But questions remained. Did they all need a CT scan? And if it was negative, did they even need to be admitted? It will be hard for many to understand the importance and impact of this line of investigation as most of these patients no longer come to the attention of the trauma service but are often treated and released by our emergency medicine colleagues.

The study in question was performed to help answer these questions. It was crafted by the first dedicated multicenter trauma trials group in response to smaller, single center studies[1] (Reference #7 of the paper). While there is no doubt that retrospective studies have inherent limitations, this study should serve as a model for how to minimize the deficiencies. First, the authors met and developed a schema and common taxonomy. They performed an *a priori* power analysis to determine the number of subjects required and continued the study to ensure that number was met. While looking back 25 years, their conclusions are hardly surprising. They lent significant weight and credence to what had been identified in the earlier single center studies. The major findings are well articulated and continue to form the basis of modern treatment of minimal head injury: (1) all patients with a documented loss of consciousness should undergo cranial CT scanning; (2) patients with a normal neurologic examination and normal CT scan never need a craniotomy for intracranial pathology; and (3) a large percentage of patients admitted for neurologic observation, especially those not admitted to an ICU, are not observed.

The one limitation not examined by this study was the CT scanner itself. The study does not list the model and generation of the scanners used in the eight centers, but the time frame of the study, 1988–1991, predated the leap to helical CT scanning. Despite these data and due to the likely retrospective design and limitations of the CT technology, many physicians and neurosurgeons were still uncomfortable with the concept of discharging patients with a negative CT. The specter of patients from the pre-CT imaging era with undetected rapidly expanding epidural hematoma (EDH) or subdural hematoma (SDH) still held sway over many providers, and there continued to be an almost irrational fear of litigation from late neurologic deterioration. It would not be until a decade later in the post-helical CT era, when a prospective study of the same population identified that discharge without admission for neurologic observation was safe.[2] There is no doubt that research to change practice is difficult and progresses often too slowly. This work by Shackford and the WTA multicenter trials groups played an important, pivotal step in our current management of patients with minimal head injury.

REFERENCES

1. Livingston DH, Loder PA, Koziol J, Hunt CD. The use of CT scanning to triage patients requiring admission following minimal head injury. *J Trauma*. 1991; 31: 483–487.
2. Livingston DH, Lavery RF, Passannante MR, Skurnick JH, Baker S, Fabian TC, Fry DE, Malangoni MA. Emergency department discharge of patients with a negative cranial computed tomography scan after minimal head injury. *Ann Surg*. 2000; 232: 126–132.

Editor Notes: These authors confirmed the value of a normal head CT to exclude the need for intervention (and therefore hospital admission) in adults with minor head injury and a GCS of 15. While others had suggested these findings previously, this large multicenter retrospective review established the accuracy of the CT to identify relevant traumatic head injury patients requiring further care. The study also demonstrated the need for careful assessment and monitoring of patients with minimal head injury, as 20% required treatment.

Limitations:

Retrospective review;
Multicenter variability in patient management;
Limited long-term follow-up data.

CHAPTER 14

The Role of Secondary Brain Injury in Determining Outcome from Severe Head Injury

Chesnut RM, Marshall LF, Klauber MR, Blunt BA, Baldwin N, Eisenberg HM, Jane JA, Marmarou A, Foulkes MA. J Trauma 34(2):216–222, 1993

Abstract   As triage and resuscitation protocols evolve, it is critical to determine the major extracranial variables influencing outcome in the setting of severe head injury. We prospectively studied the outcome from severe head injury (GCS score $\leq$ 8) in 717 cases in the Traumatic Coma Data Bank. We investigated the impact on outcome of hypotension (SBP < 90 mmHg) and hypoxia ($PaO_2 \leq$ 60 mmHg or apnea or cyanosis in the field) as secondary brain insults, occurring from injury through resuscitation. Hypoxia and hypotension were independently associated with significant increases in morbidity and mortality from severe head injury. Hypotension was profoundly detrimental, occurring in 34.6% of these patients and associated with a 150% increase in mortality. The increased morbidity and mortality related to severe trauma to an extracranial organ system appeared primarily attributable to associated hypotension. Improvements in trauma care delivery over the past decade have not markedly altered the adverse influence of hypotension. Hypoxia and hypotension are common and detrimental secondary brain insults. Hypotension, particularly, is a major determinant of outcome from severe head injury. Resuscitation protocols for brain injured patients should assiduously avoid hypovolemic shock on an absolute basis.

Author Commentary by Randall M. Chesnut

This paper's origins lie in the seminal work of Professor Douglas Miller from Edinburgh, who had described the impact of early secondary insults on outcome from traumatic brain injury (TBI). For a chapter on TBI, I queried the Traumatic Coma Data Bank database to update Prof. Miller's work. The initial analysis confirmed the negative influence of early hypoxia and hypotension on outcome but was non-exclusionary (e.g., hypoxic patients could also be hypotensive). When we re-ran the analysis looking at isolated hypoxia and hypotension, it became apparent that hypotension was exceptionally and strongly correlated with worse recovery. A single measurement of a systolic blood pressure $\leq$ 90 mmHg from the injury site through arrival at the emergency department was correlated with a doubling of mortality (to 50%) and much greater morbidity, controlling for overall injury severity and other outcome predictors. Moreover, such had occurred in 34.6% of study patients. Isolated hypoxia was also detrimental but much less influential than hypotension, although the combination raised mortality to 57%.

At the time of this analysis, the practice in TBI was to restrict fluids. Any tendency toward hypervolemia was held to increase intracranial pressure (ICP). Intravenous resuscitation fluids, which otherwise would have been wide open, were "to keep open (TKO'd)." Furthermore, systemic hypertension was also avoided, again for ICP reasons. These philosophies combined with the common use of osmotic diuretics for ICP control/prophylaxis resulted in the average TBI patient being hypovolemic and frequently skirting blood pressures near hypotension. In addition to the risk of cerebral ischaemia, the vasodilation related to low cerebral perfusion pressure (CPP; [mean arterial pressure] – [intracranial pressure]) can exacerbate intracranial hypertension in patients with intact cerebral pressure autoregulation.

This paper was extremely well received by the trauma community, particularly trauma surgeons. Although far from a definitive study, the lack of evidence supporting the longstanding practice of "keeping TBI patients dry" and the desirability of volume resuscitation in polytrauma victims led to rapid and widespread abandonment of fluid restriction in TBI. The only special consideration for multiple-injury patients with a brain trauma was to use isotonic resuscitation fluids, recognizing the slightly hypotonic nature of Ringer's lactate.

Of course, as often obtains, the pendulum then swung vigorously in the opposite direction. For a decade, the concept of maintaining an acceptable CPP was skewed toward supranormal CPP targets. Published case series targeting values as high as 90 mmHg. This was finally moderated by a trial comparing ICP-based treatment to CPP-based treatment, wherein the outcomes of the two groups were similar. ICP patients died of their brain injuries; CPP patients died of complications of prolonged hypervolaemia and vasopressor use. Target CPP values were subsequently rationalized to the current credo of full isotonic resuscitation to maintain CPP values around 60 mmHg.

If there is one more general point illustrated by this paper, it is that it reinforces the value of restoring and maintaining the normal *mileau internale*, as opposed to the apparently attractive but generally misguided concept of taking physiologic values to extremes. More is not always better.

Expert Commentary by Suresh "Mitu" Agarwal

Although the mortality and morbidity of severe traumatic brain injury (Glasgow Coma Score of less or equal to 8 at presentation) remains unacceptably high, Chesnut et al. in their landmark paper were able to demonstrate that the guided efforts of clinicians to alter outcomes was possible, at least having a structured protocol to avoid hypotension and hypoxia was necessary. Modifying behavior and improving safety equipment was the purvey of the public health and injury prevention sector; however, the concept of secondary brain injury was introduced into the medical vernacular.

In particular, the use of hypovolemic resuscitation for the treatment of severe brain injured patients was derided in this multi-institutional study as the data examined from four institutions demonstrated that even one episode of hypotension, as defined as a systolic blood pressure of less than 90, would lead to an increase in mortality rate of 150%. Similarly, any episode of hypoxia, as defined as a Partial Pressure of Oxygen of less than 60, nearly doubled the mortality rate. If a patient experienced both hypoxia and hypotension, the mortality rate nearly tripled.

The impact of these findings has had a profound impact upon management of this complex group of patients. Whereas the goal prior to publication and adoption of the findings was to minimize crystalloid and volume resuscitation in order to "dry" the brain and minimize elevations in intracerebral pressure, clinicians saw the detriment of this strategy as harmful and became wary of Mannitol administration prior to adequate volume resuscitation, thereby minimizing the chance of hypotension. Subsequently, the use of hypertonic saline in the resuscitation of hypovolemic severely traumatic brain injured patients has become accepted as a modality.

The concept of prevention of secondary brain injury has led to the examination of multiple different aspects in the management of traumatic brain injury patients. The use of decompressive craniectomy, hypothermia, hypocarbia, and steroids, in addition to several other factors and therapeutics, have been studied rigorously. Interestingly, maintaining "normal" parameters, rather than aggressive intervention, has usually been found to be more effective in preventing mortality and morbidity.

Most importantly, this paper has had a significant impact upon the impetus to develop guidelines and evidence-based protocols for the management of severe TBI patients. Most notably, the Brain Trauma Foundation has established guidelines for the management of several aspects of traumatic brain injury; most recently updated in 2016. Now traumatologists throughout the world have frequently updated evidence-based rationale for their management strategies.

Chesnut et al. supported the Hippocrates tenant of "First, do no harm" in this paper and challenged the immediacy of the Monro-Kellie Doctrine by demonstrating that hypovolemic shock and hypoxia had short and long-term repercussion in this population. Armed with this evidence, preventing hypotension and hypoxia has allowed clinicians to abide by Hippocrates's aphorism.

Editor Notes: This paper demonstrated the importance of physiologic factors in the development of secondary brain injury. From the Traumatic Coma Data bank, 717 patients with severe trauma brain injury (GCS < 9) were analyzed and found to have a higher mortality if they experienced either hypotension or hypoxia. As fluid restriction with the attendant risk of hypoperfusion was commonplace at that time, this study helped to liberalize the use of fluids in resuscitation of brain injury.

Limitations:

Retrospective analysis;
Trauma databank data;
Inability to exclude the cause of hypotension or hypoxia from that specific event (presumably whatever caused the hypotension or hypoxia would have an impact on outcome);
Failure to show that it was possible to avoid the circumstance that led to the hypoxia or hypotension.

CHAPTER 15

Clearing the Cervical Spine in Multiple Trauma Victims: A Time-Effective Protocol Using Helical Computed Tomography

Nuñez Jr DB, Coin CG, LeBlang S, Becerra JL, Henry R,
Lentz K, Quencer RM. Emerg Radiol 1:273, 1994

Abstract This study was performed to evaluate helical computed tomography (HCT) as the primary method of initial cervical spine assessment in multiple trauma victims. Prospective evaluation of the cervical spine using HCT and plain film radiography (PFR) was performed in 800 patients with suspected multisystem injuries. With HCT, an average of 32 slices were obtained at 5-mm intervals from the base of the skull to T1 using helical acquisition and a bone algorithm. HCT was performed following cross-table lateral radiographs of the cervical spine in all patients. We compared HCT and PFR for detection of abnormalities and duration of examination and compared HCT with conventional CT in a subset of patients (N = 20) for image quality/lesion detectability.

Sixty-eight fractures were identified in 46 patients. HCT prospectively identified 67 fractures (98.5%), and plain films demonstrated 29 fractures (43%). No difference in image quality/lesion detectability was encountered when comparing HCT to conventional CT. HCT of the cervical spine could be completed in 4.5 minutes and added an average of only 8 minutes to the stay of the patient in the CT room. During the time of the study, the overall patient disposition time from the trauma resuscitation area was reduced from 6.5 to 4.5 hours. Rapid and accurate evaluation of the cervical spine is possible with HCT and is recommended as part of the initial imaging protocol in multiple trauma patients.

Author Commentary by Diego B. Nuñez

In the early 1990s, there was no consensus regarding the best way to deal with one of the most debated aspects of trauma care, "clearing" the cervical spine. A variety of protocols had been proposed that comprised different combinations of radiographs without or with single section CT as an adjunct for patients with equivocal plain film examinations.

In our institution, we identified significant delay in cervical spine clearance when we relied exclusively on plain films or when a combination of radiography and limited CT was used. We were frequently confronted with the scenario of repeating multiple radiographs before failing to clear the cervical spine. This failure prompted recommendation for CT examination after the majority of these patients had already undergone CT of the brain, chest, or abdomen to evaluate other injuries. As a result, double utilization of the CT scanner became frequent. Our level I trauma center receives a preselected group of high-risk patients who meet multitrauma criteria according to state regulations. Patients are classified as high risk when they meet one of several criteria, which are based on mechanism of trauma, associated injuries, and mental status. At the time, single-section CT had become an integral part of the initial evaluation of these patients, mainly to assess for cerebral or abdominal injuries, and volumetric CT had just been introduced into clinical practice. Taking advantage of the helical configuration of the ER/Trauma dedicated CT scanner installed at the University of Miami Trauma Center, we decided to prospectively evaluate the feasibility of including helical CT of the entire cervical spine in all patients meeting high-risk criteria. The hypothesis was based on two basic premises. First, this practice would allow for a faster clearance of the cervical spine and expedite patient management with improved disposition from the admitting trauma area. Second, it would allow comparison of fracture detection rate with the established practice of radiography and show that significant cervical spine injuries can be missed by plain films.

Our prospective evaluation in 800 patients showed that a significant reduction on patient trauma work-up and disposition time was obtained when cervical helical CT was offered as a screening tool rather than as a segment-limited complementary examination.

The study also determined that CT detected an important number of fractures that were not shown by radiography. This work led to additional publications from our center that highlighted that cervical spine injuries, deemed clinically significant, could be missed by radiography. These injuries included cases with neurologic, vascular, or airway abnormalities and patients with fractures considered unstable or with potential for neurologic injury.

Over the years, with additional evidence of the benefits of this practice by several authors, screening helical CT of the cervical spine became established as an integral part of the initial trauma imaging work-up and is considered the standard of care in emergency and trauma centers across the nation. The American College of Radiology Appropriateness Criteria Guidelines recommends helical CT as the most appropriate imaging examination for suspected cervical spine trauma.

Expert Commentary by Natasha Keric

The start of the paper reads, "Clearing the cervical spine in multiple trauma victims remains a challenging and controversial issue." It is fascinating that, two decades later, this statement still holds true, despite this revolutionary study, which advanced the practice of evaluating trauma patients with possible cervical spine injury using CT scanning.

To put it in perspective, before the use of CT, plain films were the standard of care in imaging the cervical spine. CT scans at the time were still new, costly, took time to "warm up" and reformat, and were only used as a complementary modality. Plain film series included a cross-table lateral, anteroposterior, odontoid, and occasionally a swimmer's radiographic view. Time to obtain adequate views with plain films usually required multiple repeated images and took 15 minutes at minimum with the most ideal of circumstances (in a cooperative patient). In actuality, the average time for imaging was usually about 25 minutes. Plain films still did not permit the clinician to visualize the entire lateral cervical spine 25% of the time; 20% of the fractures were unstable C1 and C2 fractures; and 61% of cervical fractures were missed. This delay in diagnosis is hard to fathom in today's age of information technology where images are available to us in a matter of seconds. This study led to an era of efficiency, safety, and quality in managing trauma patients with a possible cervical spine injury.

Nuñez and colleagues found that using a helical CT scan (32 slices with 5-mm intervals from base of skull to T1), 98.5% of fractures can be detected (versus 43% using plain films). This was superior to plain films for demonstration of injuries specifically at the craniocervical junction, C1-C2 and C6-T1 segments, and added only 4.5 minutes to the total CT examination. This protocol translated to not only a reduction in patient disposition from 6.5 to 4.5 hours in the trauma resuscitation area, but a more accurate and rapid evaluation of multiple trauma patients.

Since this study, the pendulum has swung with CT scans evolving into high efficiency multislice detectors, and became the primary imaging modality for screening trauma patients with sensitivity and negative predictive values approaching 100% for clinically significant cervical spine injuries.

Even with supportive data, the idea of using CT scanning for screening cervical spine injury has continued to spur debate and research in today's practice. Several multicenter trials (1–3) have brought to light controversial topics such as: evaluating an obtunded patient with a CT scan alone; the risk of missing a ligamentous injury; the benefits of routine use of MRI as an adjunctive tool;

defining what degree of degenerative disease can still be considered a normal CT; and what to do with a patient who has a negative CT of the cervical spine with a high clinical index of suspicion. Challenging and controversial indeed!

REFERENCES

1. Como JJ, Diaz JJ, Dunham CM, et al. Practice management guidelines for identification of cervical spine injuries following trauma: Update from the eastern association for the surgery of trauma practice management guidelines committee. *J Trauma.* 2009; 67(3): 651–659.
2. Patel M, Humble SS, Cullinane DC, et al. Cervical spine collar clearance in the obtunded adult trauma patient: A systematic review and practice management guideline for the Eastern Association for the Surgery of Trauma. *J Trauma Acute Care Surg.* 2015; 78(2): 430–441.
3. Inaba K, Byerly S, Bush LD, et al. Cervical spine clearance: A prospective Western Trauma Association Multi-institutional Trial. *J Trauma Acute Care Surg.* 2016; 81(6): 1122–1130.

Editor Notes: The routine use of helical CT to assess the cervical spine was proposed in this study. Helical CT was shown to be highly accurate and comparable to conventional CT and much better than plain films in this comparative trial of 800 patients. In addition to being extremely accurate (identifying 67 or 68 fractures), the helical CT added only an average of 8 minutes to the CT room stay. Overall time in the emergency center was substantially reduced.

Limitations:

None;
In fact, this study would be likely even more impressive today with the higher quality CT technology.

CHAPTER 16

Penetrating Neck Injuries: Helical CT Angiography for Initial Evaluation

Múnera F, Soto JA, Palacio DM, Castañeda J, Morales C, Sanabria A, Gutiérrez JE, García G. Radiology 224(2):366–372, 2002

Abstract   The effects of Múnera and colleagues' landmark work on the utilization of new technology for an old problem has been profound. For the trauma surgeon who cares for a substantial number of patients with penetrating injuries to the neck, Múnera and colleagues' prospective study utilizing helical CT angiography in hemodynamically stable patients showing a sensitivity of 100%, a specificity of 98%, and positive predictive value of 93% and a negative predictive value of 100% changed the way things were done. It helped by improving both patient outcomes by decreasing the rate of unnecessary neck explorations and their inevitable complications and by freeing up surgeons' time for more productive pursuits.

Purpose   To report an experience with helical computed tomographic (CT) angiography as the initial procedure to rule out arterial lesions caused by penetrating neck injuries.

Materials and Methods   Over 27 months, 175 patients were referred for helical CT angiography of the neck because of clinical suspicion of arterial injuries. The protocol included a 100-mL bolus of nonionic contrast material injected at 4.5 mL/sec, with 11-second scanning delay, 3-mm collimation, and pitch of 1.3–2.0. CT images were interpreted prospectively by the emergency radiologist, and two radiologists retrospectively interpreted studies with consensus. Outcome was determined with examination of patients and their charts. The sensitivity, specificity, and positive and negative predictive values were calculated.

Results   Studies in two patients were considered inadequate for diagnosis; these patients were referred for conventional arteriography and had normal findings. In 27 patients (15.6%), arterial lesions were detected. One patient had two arterial injuries. Lesions demonstrated with helical CT angiography were arterial occlusion (n = 14), pseudoaneurysm (n = 8), pseudoaneurysm and arteriovenous fistulae (n = 4), and partial thrombosis (n = 2). The remaining 146 patients had normal arteries. On the basis of these findings, patients were treated with surgery (n = 21), endovascular intervention (n = 7), and observation alone (n = 146).

Conclusions   Results indicate that helical CT angiography can be used as the initial method for evaluation in patients with possible arterial injuries of the neck.

Author Commentary by Felipe Múnera

It is generally agreed that hemodynamically unstable patients and those with "hard signs" of vascular or aerodigestive tract injury, are immediately taken for surgical exploration with endovascular techniques, now sometimes used as an adjunct in the management of these patients. However, managing penetrating neck trauma in hemodynamically stable patients without clinical signs requiring mandatory exploration has been fraught with controversy.

Before the carefully designed paper by Weight in 1987, the risk of missing an esophageal injury was often used as a justification for mandatory neck exploration. This prospective study using surgical exploration as the gold standard provided further evidence for selective management of patients with penetrating injuries who did not have a clinical indication for immediate exploration. Based in part on Weight's data, stable patients with penetrating neck injuries without hard clinical signs were initially evaluated with arteriography and esophagogram or endoscopy. This approach remained as the most accepted management algorithm for many years.

In 2000, we published our first manuscript using CT angiogram (CTA) to evaluate patients with penetrating neck injuries. When I finished my training in the United States, I went back to my native Colombia for a few years, and we published a series of papers on the use of CTA to evaluate for penetrating neck injuries. Our first manuscript was a prospective study of 60 patients who had injuries in various zones and CTA was compared to conventional 4-vessel angiography. CTA was 90% sensitive and 100% specific for detecting vascular injury. This corresponded to a 100% positive-predictive value and 98% negative-predictive value. Only a common carotid artery pseudoaneurysm that was not included in the CTA field of view was missed. This was followed by a prospective series of 175 patients comparing CTA to conventional angiography, surgery, and clinical outcome. CTA had a 100% sensitivity, 98.6% specificity, 92.8% positive-predictive value, and 100% negative-predictive value.[1-3]

Over the last couple of decades, CTA became the initial study of choice for evaluating vascular and aerodigestive injuries as many additional authors reported similar results. Nevertheless, the original paper by Weight still has relevance as patients with trajectories suspicious for possible esophageal injury without direct CT evidence of injury may still need to be evaluated with an esophagogram and/or esophagoscopy.

REFERENCES

1. Múnera F, Soto JA, Palacio D, et al. Diagnosis of arterial injuries caused by penetrating trauma to the neck: Comparison of helical CT angiography and catheter angiography. *Radiology*. 2000; 216: 356–362.
2. Múnera F, Soto JA, Palacio DM, et al. Helical CTA for the initial evaluation of penetrating neck injuries. *Radiology*. 2002; 224: 366–372.
3. Múnera F, Cohn S, Rivas LA. Penetrating injuries of the neck: Use of helical computed tomographic angiography. *J Trauma*. 2005; 58(2): 413–418.

Expert Commentary by Peter A. Burke

Penetrating injuries of the neck are difficult at best. Nowhere else but the neck are so many vital structures from all major embryological systems, aerodigestive, neurovascular, in such close proximity with little or no intrinsic anatomic protection. Historically, the treatment of penetrating neck injuries has evolved, and the 2002 paper by Múnera and colleagues represents a major innovation and a significant enhancement and adaption in this evolutionary pathway. Before World War II, penetrating neck injuries were treated with a watch and wait approach. This resulted in a mortality rate as high as 35%.[1] It was then replaced by the adoption of a mandatory surgical exploration of all penetrating neck injuries. While this evolution improved and mortality, it led to high rates of nontherapeutic surgical exploration, as high as 53%,[2] with the inevitable negative effects on resource utilization, surgeons' time, and costs. In response to this, in the mid-1990s, the next modification to the treatment of penetrating neck injuries was a variation on the mandatory surgical exploration theme involving a zone-based approach for stable patients with such injuries. While still holding to the concept that all penetrating neck injury patients should be explored but given the anatomic difficulties in exploring Zone 1 and Zone 3 and the relative ease and safety of exploring Zone 2, a practice of exploring Zone 2 injuries while watching Zones 1 and 3 was adopted. This then led to a decrease in negative explorations overall, but Zone 2 injuries were still being explored unnecessarily utilizing scarce resources, time, and costs. Research into which approach was best varied with studies showing that outcomes were equivocal between mandatory exploration and watching and waiting of Zone 2 injuries, and EAST practice guidelines concluded that both were safe.[3,4]

However, it was not until advancements in imaging technology, such as the helical and multidetector CT scanners, were brought to bear that a no-zone strategy for stable patients with penetrating neck injuries was truly adopted. Múnera and collaborators utilized this advance in technology in a robust population of penetrating neck injury patients and showed that helical CT angiography could be safely and effectively used in stable patients at risk for vascular injuries in the neck. Múnera and collaborators' paper published in 2002 changed the way trauma surgeons approached stable patients with penetrating neck injuries and that validity of their results for the most part has been borne out over time and by the experience of others. With any change brought on by new technology, there are downsides. CT angiography is most robust at imaging the vasculature, but the neck contains many other important structures whose integrity may be more difficult to ascertain with CT. This is probably most true for the esophagus, and it must be remembered that potential injuries to the esophagus must be effectively pursued and ruled out. CT angiography also requires complex equipment and technical expertise and when unavailable, older, perhaps less elegant means, must be employed to rule out injury. With any significant change, there will be an unforeseen consequence. For instance, if we do not routinely explore Zone 2 injuries, how will we provide the experience needed to teach the next generation? While there is some abstract validity to this fear, it becomes more incumbent on us to find alternative methods to provide this experience to the next generation, and not to deprive the patient of the advantages of new and better ways of diagnosing injury. Múnera and colleagues' paper illustrates the advantage of new techniques that can be brought to bear for improved patient care. Technology, regardless of whether you believe it is good or bad, brings on change and is an evolutionary force. So be prepared, clinical care will continue to change, and it is our responsibility to ensure it is for the better.

REFERENCES

1. Thal ER, Meyer DM. Penetrating neck trauma. *Curr Probl Surg*. 1992; 29: 1.
2. Apffelstaedt JP, Muller R. Results of mandatory exploration for penetrating neck trauma. *World J Surg*. 1994; 18: 917.
3. Tisherman SA, Bokhari F. Collier B, et al. Clinical practice guideline: Penetrating zone II neck trauma. *J Trauma*. 2008; 64: 1392.
4. Penetrating Neck Injuries: Initial evaluation and management, Kim Newton, Up To Date 2017, Wolters Kluwer. Peter A. Burke, MD, FACS Chief of Trauma Services, Boston Medical Center Chief of Acute Care & Trauma Surgery, Boston Medical Center Professor of Surgery, Boston University School of Medicine, Boston Medical Center, Boston, MA.

Editor Notes: This was an important study that found that CT angiogram of the neck was effective in identifying arterial injuries when compared with conventional arteriography. 15.6% (27/173) patients had the diagnosis of arterial injuries of the neck.

Limitations:

All patients did not have a neck exploration or a selective angiogram, therefore some injuries could have been missed;
The study is limited by artifact caused by metal foreign bodies.

CHAPTER 17

Blunt Cerebrovascular Injury Screening with 32-Channel Multidetector Computed Tomography: More Slices Still Don't Cut It

DiCocco JM, Emmett KP, Fabian TC, Zarzaur BL, Williams JS, Croce MA. Ann Surg 253(3):444–450, 2011

Abstract Until the mid-1990s, blunt cerebrovascular injuries (BCVIs) were considered a rare (1 in 1,000 blunt trauma admissions), but devastating injury, diagnosed on the basis of neurologic signs and symptoms that were unexplained by head and c-spine CT. In 1996, a seminal paper by Fabian and colleagues[1] changed the landscape. Vigilant clinical evaluation and early cervical arteriography led to the diagnosis in an incredible 0.7% of their blunt trauma patients. In addition, they demonstrated improved neurologic outcomes with systemic anticoagulation.

Objective We sought to determine the diagnostic accuracy of computed tomographic angiography (CTA) using 32-channel multidetector computed tomography for blunt cerebrovascular injuries (BCVIs).

Background Unrecognized BCVI is a cause of stroke in young trauma patients. Digital subtraction angiography (DSA), the reference standard, is invasive, expensive, and time-consuming. CTA has been rapidly adopted by many institutions because of its availability, less resource intensive, and noninvasive nature. However, conflicting results comparing CTA and DSA have been reported. Studies with 16-channel CTA report a wide range of sensitivities for BCVI diagnosis.

Methods From January 2007 through May 2009, patients with risk factors for BCVI underwent both CTA and DSA. All CTAs were performed using a 32-channel multidetector CT scanner. Using DSA as the reference standard, the diagnostic accuracy of CTA for determination of BCVI was calculated.

Results There were 684 patients who met the inclusion criteria. Ninety patients (13%) had 109 injuries identified; 52 carotid and 57 vertebral injuries were diagnosed. CTA failed to detect 53 confirmed BCVI, yielding a sensitivity of 51%.

Conclusion Given the devastation of stroke and high mortality from missed injuries, this study demonstrates that even with more advanced technology (32- vs. 16-channel), CTA is inadequate for BCVI screening. Digital subtraction angiography remains the gold standard for the diagnosis of BCVI.

Author Commentary by Martin A. Croce

Blunt cerebrovascular injuries (BCVIs) were once thought to be relatively rare injuries. It was noted that some patients, especially young patients, developed unexplained strokes resulting in severe disability or death. Further investigation identified BCVI in these patients. A number of studies were published, many from Memphis and Denver, which led to widespread screening for this devastating injury. With this screening, BCVI is now identified in approximately 2% of blunt trauma patients. While it is clear that screening is beneficial, the modality used for screening is debatable.

All things being equal, the optimal screening test would be digital subtraction angiography (DSA). It is the reference standard for diagnosis and management. DSA is invasive and requires 24 hours of cerebral angiographic availability, so other screening methods were described. The most accepted identified patients with significant trauma to the head, face, and neck (cervical spine fracture, skull base fracture, Le Fort fracture, unexplained neurologic deficit). Patients with these injuries would undergo DSA, and DSA in this population identified approximately 80% of the injuries.

Many institutions adopted computed tomographic angiography (CTA) for BCVI screening since it is less invasive and much less resource intensive than DSA. This rapid adoption of CTA as a screening test for BCVI occurred without rigorous testing, however. The few studies that were used to justify a 16-channel CTA had wide ranges of sensitivity. It is likely that there were patients who had missed BCVI, but screening CTA continued. Those with adverse outcomes from missed BCVI were likely thought to have suffered from worsening associated brain injuries, and unexpected deaths were probably thought to be due to myocardial infarction or pulmonary embolus. Since the injury is uncommon, the real impact of missed injuries would most likely be noticed primarily in high volume trauma centers.

This study set out to see if the newer generation (at that time) of CT scanners would be an appropriate screening test. It was the first to include a large number of patients (684) who had *both* CTA and DSA, and the data was critically analyzed. The CTA was performed with a 32-slice scanner. All blunt trauma patients who were receiving a CT of the head due to their trauma also underwent CTA and DSA. Performance of CTA and DSA was not dependent of the presence or absence of the standard head/face/neck injury criteria. Compared to DSA, CTA was found to have a sensitivity of 51%, specificity of 97%, a positive predictive value of 43%, and a negative predictive value of 98%. It was concluded that CTA alone was inadequate as a definitive screening test for patients at risk for BCVI.

This study did identify an important benefit of CTA. As the previous studies showed that approximately 80% of BCVI were associated with other injuries about the head and neck, an additional 16% of BCVI were identified using the criteria of CTA for all patients receiving a CT of the head. Thus, the 32-slice CTA had more utility as a screening *criterion* than as a screening *test*.

Expert Commentary by Walter L. Biffl

It had long been suspected that many injuries were clinically occult, and it followed that early diagnosis and treatment might reduce the morbidity and mortality of BCVI-related stroke. In 1998, our group in Denver reported the first study of liberal screening of asymptomatic patients (in the 1996 Memphis paper, over 90% of patients were symptomatic).[2] Arteriography was performed based on injury mechanisms and patterns, rather than signs and symptoms of ischemic neurologic insults. Injuries were found in 1% of blunt trauma patients, and three-quarters of them were asymptomatic at diagnosis.

Not surprisingly, the trauma community was initially skeptical. The notion of performing invasive arteriography, which often required transfer to a level I trauma center, and systemically anticoagulating trauma patients was considered heretical. But awareness of BCVI was increasing. Noninvasive diagnosis was clearly preferable for a number of reasons, but the Denver and Memphis groups both published studies in 2002 finding that neither CT nor MR angiography (CTA, MRA) offered acceptable diagnostic accuracy.[3,4] But these studies were performed with early generation CT scanners, and over the next several years different groups reported that multidetector-row CT (MDCT) was actually quite good. With liberal screening, centers were reporting 1% or higher incidence of BCVI, with no clinically important injuries missed by 16-channel MDCT.[5-7] Screening protocols were becoming widespread, and BCVI were being diagnosed at unprecedented rates.

A few investigators reported on the inaccuracies of CTA.[8-10] The paper selected by the editors was one of those. While the broader trauma community had embraced CTA for BCVI screening, the Memphis group continued to rigorously compare CTA and arteriography. They cautioned about missing higher-grade injuries of clinical significance. While this was an important lesson, the question in many people's minds was, "What now?" Were we really going to go back to invasive arteriography in everybody? In the end, most centers stuck with their institutional protocols and used MDCT for diagnosis. This probably resulted in fewer missed injuries than if it had been abandoned; clinicians would likely have been much more selective in their screening.

The Memphis group deserves a great deal of credit for paving the way and shaping the diagnostic approach and treatment of BCVI. And with their 2014 proclamation that "64 slices finally cut it," CTA is here to stay.[11]

REFERENCES

1. Fabian TC, Patton JH Jr, Croce MA, et al. Blunt carotid injury: Importance of early diagnosis and anticoagulant therapy. *Ann Surg*. 1996; 223: 513.
2. Biffl WL, Moore EE, Ryu RK, et al. The unrecognized epidemic of blunt carotid arterial injuries: Early diagnosis improves neurologic outcome. *Ann Surg*. 1998; 228: 462.
3. Biffl WL, Ray CE Jr, Moore EE, et al. Noninvasive diagnosis of blunt cerebrovascular injuries: A preliminary report. *J Trauma*. 2002; 53: 850.
4. Miller PR, Fabian TC, Croce MA, et al. Prospective screening for blunt cerebrovascular injuries: Analysis of diagnostic modalities and outcomes. *Ann Surg*. 2002; 236: 386.
5. Berne JD, Reuland KS, Villarreal DH, et al. Sixteen-slice multi-detector computed tomographic angiography improves the accuracy of screening for blunt cerebrovascular injury. *J Trauma*. 2006; 60: 1204.
6. Biffl WL, Egglin T, Benedetto B, et al. Sixteen-slice computed tomographic angiography is a reliable noninvasive screening test for clinically significant blunt cerebrovascular injuries. *J Trauma*. 2006; 60: 745.
7. Eastman AL, Chason DP, Perez CL, et al. Computed tomographic angiography for the diagnosis of blunt cervical vascular injury: Is it ready for primetime? *J Trauma*. 2006; 60: 925.
8. Utter GH, Hollingworth W, Hallam DK, et al. Sixteen-slice CT angiography in patients with suspected blunt carotid and vertebral artery injuries. *J Am Coll Surg*. 2006; 203: 838.
9. Malhotra AK, Camacho M, Ivatury RR, et al. Computed tomographic angiography for the diagnosis of blunt carotid/vertebral artery injury: A note of caution. *Ann Surg*. 2007; 246: 632.
10. Goodwin RB, Beery PR 2nd, Dorbish RJ, et al. Computed tomographic angiography versus conventional angiography for the diagnosis of blunt cerebrovascular injury in trauma patients. *J Trauma*. 2009; 67: 1046.
11. Paulus EM, Fabian TC, Savage SA, et al. Blunt cerebrovascular injury screening with 64-channel multidetector computed tomography: More slices finally cut it. *J Trauma Acute Care Surg*. 2014; 76: 279.

Editor Notes: The accuracy of the CT angiography study for identifying patients with blunt cerebrovascular injury was tested in this elegant investigation. Nearly 700 patients were studied prospectively with both 32-channel CT scan and digital subtraction angiography (gold standard) over a 30-month time period. The CT scan failed to identify about half of the lesions detected by angiogram. The study suggested that CT angiography is not an effective screening tool for blunt cerebrovascular injury. Considering that this has been used to exclude this injury for a number of years, it made clinicians reconsider the importance (if any) of blunt cerebrovascular injury as it appears that about half of lesions have been missing without apparent sequelae.

Limitations:

Older technology may be inferior to the current CT scan techniques;
Of the 90 patients identified as injured, only 13 had strokes, 9 of which were present on admission, and 3 were felt to be related to treatment (anticoagulation), and the one other stroke patient died despite intervention. The indications and benefit of treatment in the other 50 patients are uncertain.

CHAPTER 18

Indications for Operation in Abdominal Trauma

Shaftan GW. Am J Surg 99:657–664, 1960

Abstract A study by one of the giants of US trauma surgery from nearly 60 years ago makes for a fascinating read by definition. There is a myriad of pearls and novel (for that era) observations, which stand true today and have lost nothing from their original value. Until then, lessons learned in previous wars were translated into civilian practice and called for early operation of all penetrating abdominal injuries. The study by Shaftan reversed this standard of care, proving that careful clinical examination and subsequent observation could distinguish those requiring an abdominal exploration from those who could be managed expectantly.

Author Commentary by Gerald W. Shaftan

This report originated because of a surgical tragedy. In 1956, a 21-year-old male arrived at the Kings County Hospital Center (KCHC) in an alcoholic stupor and with a small stab wound in the left upper quadrant. As our classic approach, he had a routine exploratory celiotomy but there was no penetration into the peritoneal cavity. Immediately on recovering from anesthesia, however, the patient went into delirium tremens and he continued in DTs despite treatment with massive intramuscular paraldehyde. On the third postoperative day, he eviscerated his midline wound and was repaired with mass stainless-steel wire suture. Still in DTs, with uncontrolled alcohol withdrawal convulsions, he eviscerated again on the seventh postoperative day, cutting a loop of small bowel on the retention sutures. This was repaired, and the wound again had a mass closure. But on the eleventh postoperative day he eviscerated a third time, cutting three loops of small bowel. He died 14 days after admission.

His death, following a therapeutically unnecessary celiotomy, prompted Dwight Spreng, my Chief Resident, and I to do a review of our 3-year past experience of 133 patients with abdominal trauma treated by the University Surgical Service at KCHC, as noted in this article. We were surprised to learn that, despite our strict departmental policy of routine exploration of patients with penetrating trauma, almost half of the patients with stab wounds were never explored, and some of the gunshot wounds also were treated without operation. This retrospective review was presented at our Morbidity and Mortality conference on December 24, 1955. Our chairman, Clarence Dennis, firmly believed in routine exploration of abdominal injury, although he had little experience with penetrating injury from Minneapolis. Nevertheless, as a true scientist, he felt that we should clinically investigate "selective operation in penetrating trauma," (his words), so that on January 1, 1956, routine operation for all abdominal trauma no longer was mandated on our service at Kings County Hospital.

This presentation of the first 3 years of selective operation was not kindly received at the American Association for the Surgery of Trauma (AAST) meeting held in Mount Washington, New Hampshire, in 1959. The future editor of the nascent *Journal of Trauma* felt that I was the most dangerous surgeon in America. Gradually, especially following the paper by Nance, selective celiotomy, especially for stab wounds of the anterior abdomen and flank, became acceptable in many parts of the United States, even in Texas. In 2001, the classic paper by Velmahos and Demetriades "Selective Nonoperative Management in 1,856 Patients with Abdominal Gunshot Wounds" confirmed that gunshot wounds also could safely be handled in the same fashion. Finally, Velmahos's paper in the current *Journal of the American College of Surgeons* should leave no doubt that as I said in the conclusion to my paper, "The application of trained surgical judgment rather than dogma is the more rational and intelligent approach to the management of abdominal injury."

Expert Commentary by George C. Velmahos

In describing 180 patients with abdominal trauma of a penetrating nature in 62% of them, Dr. Shaftan informed the readership of *The American Journal of Surgery* in 1960 that operating routinely on patients with abdominal trauma was unnecessary and potentially dangerous. Despite the fact that patients with blunt abdominal trauma were included in the analysis, the study is remembered for the bold stance of managing penetrating abdominal trauma patients without an operation.

The experience of Kings County Hospital served as the springboard for other teams to practice selective management of penetrating abdominal injuries. Francis Nance from Charity Hospital in New Orleans, Thomas Berne from the LA County/USC Medical Center, and Demetrios Demetriades from the Baragwanath Hospital in South Africa published about massive series of abdominal stab wounds, which were managed safely without a routine operation. Those who had diffuse abdominal tenderness or hemodynamic instability were rushed to the operating room, while the rest were observed under careful protocols of repeated clinical exams and in-house monitoring. Slowly, the concept spilled over to abdominal gunshot wounds, although it took much longer to convince the surgical world that a gunshot hole in the abdominal skin of patients without peritonitis or shock did not necessarily require a midline laparotomy. Of note, the study by Shaftan included only nine abdominal gunshot wounds, but large series from South Africa and Los Angeles in the 1990s established the concept of selective, nonoperative management for this type of injury. The concept was further validated by additional studies, showing that even in trauma centers without large penetrating trauma volumes, abdominal gunshot wounds could be managed selectively by dedicated trauma teams that used sensible protocols.

Today, the new generations of trauma surgeons find it natural to admit for observation a patient with a penetrating injury to the abdomen. Even further, assisted by computed tomography, they may feel comfortable to discharge a patient straight from the Emergency Room, if an extraperitoneal track is established. One should not forget that this current standard of care, which has saved numerous patients from harmful, emergent operations, is owed to the astute observations, clinical skills, and scientific integrity of Dr. Shaftan and his team.

Editor Notes: This was one of the seminal papers suggesting the accuracy of serial physical exams in excluding injury after penetrating abdominal trauma. Prior to that time, mandatory laparotomy was the established management protocol for these trauma victims. From 1956 to 1958, 180 consecutive patients with abdominal trauma admitted to Kings County Hospital were assessed. Nearly 70% of the patients had successful nonoperative management with only 7% undergoing nontherapeutic celiotomies.

Limitations:

Retrospective study;
Small population;
Limited data on method of serial exams and frequency;
No imaging studies;
Limited data provided regarding clinical presentation and operative findings.

CHAPTER 19

Evaluation of Abdominal Trauma by Computed Tomography

Federle MP, Goldberg HI, Kaiser JA, Moss AA, Jeffrey RB
Jr, Mall JC. Radiology 138(3):637–644, 1981

Abstract Computed tomography (CT) was used in the evaluation of 100 patients suffering abdominal trauma. The type of trauma was blunt in 78 patients, penetrating in eight, and iatrogenic in 14. Forty percent of cases had normal CT scans, while 60% showed substantial abdominal or retroperitoneal injuries. Surgery, clinical follow-up, and repeated radiologic examinations confirmed the accuracy of CT, and there were no cases in which medical or surgical management was inappropriately guided by CT. A wide variety of injuries was detected, including 19 splenic, eight hepatic, six pancreatic, 13 renal, 13 retroperitoneal or abdominal wall, and one intraperitoneal. CT has major advantages over plain radiography, radionuclide imaging, and angiography in assessment of trauma-induced injuries.

Author Commentary by Michael P. Federle

Whole body CT scanning reached the United States in 1975, and for the first few years was available mostly in large, university medical centers. While head CT had an immediate acceptance and impact on diagnosis and management of head trauma, there were only a few scattered case reports of its use to diagnose abdominal trauma. I finished my abdominal imaging fellowship in 1979 and took a faculty position at San Francisco General Hospital (SFGH), the "County" hospital affiliated with the University of California, San Francisco.

In 1979, Don Trunkey, the Chief of Surgery at SFGH published his landmark research establishing the importance of Trauma Centers in expediting and improving the care of injured patients, and SFGH became the designated major trauma center for the city and county. Jack McAninch was the Chief of Urology at SFGH and had already established himself as the pioneering expert in the management of genitourinary injuries. Together, we began evaluating the role of CT in evaluation of abdominal trauma, and I could not have asked for a more collegial and supportive group of individuals with which to work.

The paradigm for evaluation of blunt abdominal trauma, at that time, was to perform diagnostic peritoneal lavage; having instilled a liter of saline into the peritoneal cavity, one looked at fluid that was subsequently retrieved. If it was pink enough (blood-tinged) that you could not read newsprint through it, you performed a laparotomy. Many nontherapeutic laparotomies were the result, although not all surgeons would agree as to what was necessary.

Within a couple of years, we had studied our first 100 patients with CT and submitted our manuscript to *Radiology* for publication. The CT image quality was terrible, but the results were quite encouraging, as all injuries detected by CT seemed to correlate well with those found in the operating room. Keep in mind that each CT section took about 10 seconds to acquire and even longer to be reconstructed and displayed by the computer, resulting in images blurred by patient, respiratory, and peristaltic motion. The spatial resolution was about $2 \times 2 \times 10$ mm. By contrast, we now commonly perform a CT evaluation of the head, chest, abdomen, and pelvis with image acquisition and display occurring almost instantaneously as the patient is moved through the scanner, with a spatial resolution of 1 mm or less in the X, Y, and Z axes.

Drawing encouragement from our initial results and surgical colleagues, we performed ongoing studies with rapidly improving CT equipment, all the while helping to redefine the exact nature of traumatic injuries (contributing to the American Association for the Surgery of Trauma [AAST] Injury Scoring Scale) and leading to widespread acceptance of informed selection of patients for surgery, hospital surveillance, or even discharge from the emergency department. Our manuscript became one of the 100 most-cited articles in *Radiology*, and our results were corroborated by other investigators, helping to redefine the diagnosis and management of abdominal trauma.

Expert Commentary by Thomas M. Scalea

My hospital acquired its first CT scanner in the early 1980s when I was a resident. We quickly realized that this new modality would have applicability in trauma evaluation, particularly in the abdomen.

At that time, the diagnostic tests available were physical examination and diagnostic peritoneal lavage. The rate of nontherapeutic laparotomy based on either was high. As we pored over the grainy images, crude by today's standards, but revolutionary then, the ability to identify organ-specific injury, and image the retroperitoneum simultaneously revolutionized our care. For instance, prior to CT, investigating the retroperitoneum required a Gastrografin UGI and enema, as well as an IVP, studies that have essentially disappeared. Patients were then observed for 3 days, to avoid missing a retroperitoneal hollow viscus injury. How things have changed.

At that time, CT was a time-consuming exam. The scans took 10–20 minutes of scan time to complete. The head scan was done, and the patient had to be rotated 180 degrees to image the torso. As helical scans were not yet available, imaging the vasculature was impossible. The scanners heated up and had to be allowed to cool between patients. Scanners were in the radiology suites, not the ED. In Brooklyn, the scanner was one building over and three floors up. Mornings after a busy weekend night, I distinctly remember seeing patients lined up on stretchers, like train cars, outside the scanner awaiting CT. By the time the last person was scanned, it was 12 hours after injury. They had clearly triaged themselves. Taking a marginal patient to CT was forbidden. Patients had surgical exploration because they were too sick to go to CT; often those explorations were negative. We were simply terrified of having a patient die on the scanner. My mentor, Dr. Gerry Shaftan had a slide that said, "Death begins in X-Ray." I still use that slide in my talks. Early CT easily fitted in to that concept.

The authors reviewed 100 CT scans that were performed at San Francisco General Hospital and a community affiliate over nearly 2 1/2 years. If the two hospitals saw a combined 2,500 trauma patients per year, likely an underestimate, they performed CT scans in well under 5% of patients. Sixty percent of the scans were positive for injury. The use of CT scanning is now so ubiquitous it is hard to imagine a patient being evaluated without CT. The positive rate of CT scanning in my institution is under 2%. The ABCs of trauma are now airway, breathing, CT scan; far different than their practice.

Even in 1980, CT was able to diagnose the myriad of injuries in the abdomen and retroperitoneum that we still commonly see. CT detected splenic, liver, and kidney injuries, injuries to the retroperitoneum, flank, and anterior abdominal wall, and free air associated with small bowel injury. Impressively, 6% of the injuries identified were pancreatic, an injury that is even now subtle on CT. CT was able to accurately characterize injuries identifying lacerations, subcapsular hematomas, and associated hemoperitoneum.

In all 40 patients with a negative CT scan, there were no missed injuries. The authors also identified the role of serial CTs, the use of CT to identify post injury/operative complications, and the role CT can play in preoperative planning. The authors even used CT in a few patients with penetrating trauma, years before the technique was described in detail. While injury identified on CT generally prompted open exploration, the authors did hint that CT could help in nonoperative management.

Whole body CT is now used indiscriminately, even in patients with minor mechanisms. Hitting a single key on the computer orders a whole body scan. It is fascinating to recognize that 35 years ago, not that long ago, we were just beginning the journey that has taken us to this point. We owe investigators like Federle and his colleagues a huge debt of gratitude for pointing us in this direction. Perhaps, we should relearn some of their lessons, stop a minute to appreciate their contributions, and think before mindlessly hitting that computer key again.

Editor Notes: These investigators were among the first to describe the value of abdominal CT scanning for identification of injuries in this study of 100 trauma patients. The concept of nonoperative management of abdominal injuries was further solidified by this and subsequent work.

Limitations:

Small population, lack of gold standard confirmation in all cases (only 31/60 injuries were confirmed at surgery);
Very small penetrating trauma experience.

CHAPTER 20

Prospective Evaluation of Surgeons' Use of Ultrasound in the Evaluation of Trauma Patients

Rozycki GS, Ochsner MG, Jaffin JH, Champion HR.
J Trauma 34(4):516–526; discussion 526–527, 1993

Abstract   Ultrasound diagnostic imaging has been demonstrated to be a valuable investigative tool in the evaluation of trauma patients in Europe and Japan. In the United States, however, ultrasound has not been widely used by trauma surgeons because of its lack of availability in the trauma resuscitation area and the associated cost and lack of full-time availability of a technician. In this prospective study, four attending trauma surgeons, four trauma fellows (PGY 6 and 7), and 25 surgical residents (PGY 4) at a level I trauma center were trained in specific ultrasound techniques to identify fluid in trauma patients with thoracoabdominal injuries. Their ultrasound evaluations of 476 patients demonstrated that, in 90 patients with clinically significant injuries, ultrasound imaging successfully detected injury in 71, for a 79% sensitivity. Specificity was 95.6%. We conclude that (1) surgeons can rapidly and accurately perform and interpret ultrasound examinations; and (2) ultrasound is a rapid, sensitive, specific diagnostic modality for detecting intra-abdominal fluid and pericardial effusion.

Author Commentary by Grace S. Rozycki

To appreciate the uniqueness of this paper, it is important to understand that, for decades, diagnostic peritoneal lavage (DPL) was the main adjunct for the evaluation of the patient after blunt trauma. DPL was rapid and accurate, but invasive, and its high sensitivity resulted in too many nontherapeutic laparotomies. The resolution and speed of the computed tomography (CT) scan was improving, but its location in the radiology suite was a significant drawback. There was a need for a noninvasive diagnostic test to be used by the surgeon in the trauma bay that would rapidly examine for pericardial and intra-abdominal blood. Although surgeons from Germany and Japan were using ultrasound in the trauma setting, there were no prospective studies (other than a preliminary progress report) of US surgeons using this tool in the trauma bay.

The impact of this paper was noteworthy because trauma surgeons developed a focused ultrasound examination to evaluate the patient with potential blunt or penetrating thoracoabdominal injury. The examination was based on the anatomic principle that blood would settle in the dependent areas; namely, the pericardial sac, Morison's pouch, the left upper quadrant, and pelvis. Surgeons learned the workings of the ultrasound machine and applied principles of ultrasound physics to obtain images. This was a huge accomplishment as ultrasound was not part of a surgeon's usual skill set. Further, as ultrasound machines did not have presets, it was often necessary for the surgeons to adjust the gain and depth. Over time, surgeons won the "turf wars" as this study showed that they could rapidly and accurately perform Focus Assessment with Sonography for Trauma (FAST); hence, practice boundaries blurred, as radiologists alone did not own the technology.

Although the FAST abdominal scans has some false negative results in patients with posttraumatic intra-abdominal bleeding, its accuracy in the diagnosis of hemopericardium is unparalleled. Prior to the use of ultrasound, the diagnosis of hemopericardium was usually made by an abnormally high or rising central venous pressure. With ultrasound, the sagittal view of the pericardial area easily identifies the presence or absence of blood in between the visceral and parietal layers. This often allows for a diagnosis prior to physiologic compromise.

It is hard to believe that most ultrasound companies would neither consider selling nor lending an ultrasound machine to surgeons in the early 1990s, for fear that it would compromise their fiduciary relationships with radiologists. Eventually, this changed as ultrasound companies identified a new market share and, with the input of trauma surgeons, they developed more compact, user-friendly machines and more durable transducers.

This report documented that surgeon-performed ultrasound was a rapid, noninvasive and portable diagnostic test. Early recognition of the presence or absence of blood in the pericardial sac and three dependent areas of the abdomen has had profound effects on the management of patients with truncal trauma for over 25 years.

Expert Commentary by Paula Ferrada

Point of care ultrasound (POCUS) is an irreplaceable tool for real-time assisted diagnosis. The applications of this instrument range from guiding procedures, fluid status evaluation, and diagnosing pneumothorax and bleeding in the thoracic and abdominal cavity, among others. This technology allows for immediate evaluation of the deteriorating patient by granting visualization of anatomical structures otherwise hidden from the naked eye. Because it is performed at the bedside, by the treating physician, it has a very high clinical yield, narrowing a differential diagnosis, and being of aid when guiding therapy.

In the last decade, the use of POCUS has gained credibility, and has been incorporated in the armamentarium of surgeons, anesthesiologists, emergency medicine, and critical care physicians. The use of POCUS has extended to the prehospital and nursing personnel as well.

Dr. Grace Rozycki is the pioneer in defining the role of surgeon-performed ultrasound in trauma patients. The current article is the landmark paper that transformed how we evaluate our patients using this tool. Preceding this publication, ultrasound was used in Europe and Asia to assist in the diagnosis of intra-abdominal bleeding. Just a year prior to this study, a report of the use of ultrasound to triage injuries during a mass casualty event was released by the *Journal of Trauma* (31:247, 1991). However, by the time this article was released, US surgeons remained skeptical about the issue.

This paper was presented as a plenary talk during the 52nd Annual Session of the American Association for the Surgery of Trauma in 1992. It describes in detail the technique for performing the now-called Focus Assessment with Sonography for Trauma (FAST). The author presented 476 patients with blunt and penetrating trauma admitted to a level I trauma center. These patients had a Diagnostic Peritoneal Lavage (DPL), CT scan, or surgical exploration within one hour of the ultrasound examination. They presented the results highlighting different categories: true negatives, true positives, false negatives, and false positives. Of note were the 19 false negative scans in the study. Nine of them were victims of blunt trauma, and 10 were patients with penetrating mechanism of injury. Not surprisingly, all patients with a penetrating mechanism required surgical exploration. Interestingly, from the blunt trauma patients in this group, two of them needed surgical exploration not because of the trauma itself, but as a consequence of the complications from DPL. The other patients with false negative results had injuries that with today's technology would likely undergo nonoperative treatment (low-grade hepatic or splenic lacerations).

This paper revolutionized how we think, and how we treat patients with blunt abdominal trauma. It was the start of many other papers defining the role of ultrasound to triage hypotensive patients. The introduction of this tool has undoubtedly resulted in less unnecessary invasive procedures on trauma patients, and the introduction of FAST has now evolved into more sophisticated studies that allow surgeons not only to evaluate anatomy, but also to interpret the physiological information obtained with these windows.

One of the limitations of ultrasound is that it is operator dependent. Contrary to avoiding the use of this technology because of this limitation, as surgeons we must embrace it, incorporate the teaching early in medical student and resident education, and understand it as another tool to help clinicians treat our patients. As the applications of POCUS keep growing, having surgeons involved in the process ensures we maintain a voice in how we use it. I believe strongly, this seminal work from Dr. Rozycki made the difference in getting surgeons involved as a vital component of training in the use of ultrasound in the acute setting.

Editor Notes: These authors supported two concepts: they confirmed that the accuracy of ultrasound was high in detecting thoracoabdominal injury; and surgeons could successfully perform ultrasound and could screen for the presence or absence of hemoperitoneum.

Limitations:

17/88 (19%) patients with injuries were missed on ultrasound;
Fluid in the peritoneal cavity was missed in 21%;
Inter- and intra-rater variability was not assessed.

CHAPTER 21

Subxiphoid Pericardiotomy versus Echocardiography: A Prospective Evaluation of the Diagnosis of Occult Penetrating Cardiac Injury

Jimenez E, Martin M, Krukenkamp I, Barrett J. Surgery 108(4):676–679; discussion 679–680, 1990

Abstract Diagnostic subxiphoid pericardiotomy (SP) is presently advocated for the diagnosis of occult cardiac injuries in patients with stable vital signs with juxta-cardiac-penetrating chest wounds. This approach, however, results in a reported 80% negative pericardial exploration rate. To investigate the reliability of bedside two-dimension echocardiography (2-D echo) in predicting cardiac injury as compared to SP, a prospective study was undertaken of patients with stable vital signs who were admitted with penetrating chest wounds that were located within the space bounded by the manubrium, nipples, and subcostal line. Initial evaluation of the patients with bedside 2-D echo was found to have a 96% accuracy, 97% specificity, and 90% sensitivity in predicting cardiac injury. The only false-negative findings were in a patient who consented to SP 18 hours after bedside 2-D echo was performed. The reliability of bedside 2-D echo compared to SP was not significantly different according to the kappa measure of reliability. These data suggest that bedside 2-D echo is an expeditious and reliable method to diagnose occult cardiac injuries during the initial assessment of a patient who had stable vital signs along with penetrating chest trauma. This approach may allow for the selective use of SP on patients with positive bedside 2-D echo and could eliminate unnecessary surgical procedures.

Expert Commentary by John Nagabiez

In 1990, Jimenez and colleagues demonstrated the feasibility of echocardiography in the diagnosis of occult cardiac injury in hemodynamically stable patients with penetrating wounds to the chest. A surgical resident and cardiology fellow diagnosed hemopericardium with 96% accuracy, 97% specificity, and 90% sensitivity, thereby eliminating a reported negative pericardial exploration rate of 80%. Prior to this, open subxyphoid pericardial "window" was the standard of care. This mandated general anesthesia, and in most institutions, a chaotic transport to an operating room, delaying all other diagnostic studies.

The procedure itself can be technically challenging, especially in the obese, and put patients at risk for complications, such as ventricular laceration, particularly in the absence of hemopericardium.

Echocardiographic results are both operator and patient dependent. Sonographer experience is paramount, and study quality decreases inversely with body habitus and patient compliance. One must also guard against over-estimating the quality of any given study. There is a tendency for the declaration of "negative echo" to propagate throughout the ranks of the trauma team, factitiously gathering authority by virtue of repetition, inhibiting consideration to repeat the study or explore surgically. Skepticism should be maintained if one has not witnessed the exam personally, particularly in patients who insidiously begin to exhibit subtle signs of early tamponade.

False negatives must be avoided as this can result in time and effort wasted pursuing incorrect diagnoses. Following a false negative study, reconsideration of the diagnoses of hemopericardium and even tamponade tends to be neglected, most notably in an otherwise healthy patient with stout physiologic reserve and persistent tachycardia. This error is minimized by keeping the diagnosis in mind and repeating the echo or exploring the pericardium. Trace hemopericardium is easily missed on echo but can lead to the development of pericarditis and increasing pericardial effusion or may lead to tamponade in the setting of a slow or delayed intrapericardial bleed.

False positivity in the trauma setting includes labeling a pericardial effusion as acute hemopericardium when, in fact, it is coincident and unrelated to the presenting complaint. This error may be avoided by considering the patient's medical and surgical history as well as the volume of fluid detected. In a hemo-dynamically stable patient, the larger the effusion, the more likely it is chronic, demonstrating physiologic compensation, and it is with less certainty that one may infer acute etiology. Certainly, the larger the effusion, the more likely drainage will be indicated regardless, but considering chronicity allows the trauma team the flexibility of attending to other potentially more urgent injuries rather than inappropriately prioritizing pericardial exploration.

Finally, sonographic detection of hemothorax may be misconstrued as hemo-pericardium (false positive). In contrast, when performed after chest radiograph and/or chest tube, a known hemothorax may lead the sonographer to dismiss actual hemopericardium as visualization of the hemothorax (false negative). There can be no doubt that the rudimentary skills required to detect occult hemopericardium by sonography are readily acquired by all members of the trauma team and invaluable in minimizing the incidence of unnecessary surgical intervention.

Expert Commentary by Robert C. Mackersie

The accurate, rapid diagnosis of penetrating cardiac injuries is critical to ensure optimal survival in this challenging group of patients. This paper established an important milestone in the development of diagnostic methods for penetrating cardiac injuries and initiated the movement away from the reflex use of the diagnostic pericardial window and toward the regular use of ultrasonography in the trauma resuscitation area. At the time of its publication, this was the largest study that involved patients suspected of having penetrating cardiac injuries and was conducted prospectively, with all but one patient having confirmatory pericardial window performed. The results, showing a high degree of specificity and sensitivity, were eventually validated by a number of subsequent studies of 2-D echocardiography used in this setting and confirmed that 2-D echo had a diagnostic accuracy similar to that of pericardial window. In addition to demonstrating the utility of 2-D echo in the trauma bay, this study was one of the first US publications to demonstrate, as was pointed out in the discussion by Dr. Lew Flint, the feasibility of training surgical residents to perform bedside ultrasound in the emergency department.

The diagnosis of penetrating cardiac wounds evolved substantially from the 1970s to the 1990s. The initial practice of selective operation for patients with penetrating trauma proximal to the heart, based solely on clinical signs of cardiac tamponade, was later abandoned due to the inaccuracy of this approach and the lethality of delayed diagnosis. Many centers adopted a more proactive approach using either limited thoracotomy or performing a diagnostic subxiphoid pericardial window, even in hemodynamically normal patients. This resulted in many "negative" procedures but reduced the incidence of missed injuries.

As 2-D echocardiography became more accessible in the 1980s, isolated case reports of its use in the setting of potential cardiac trauma began to appear and stimulated interest in this approach. A retrospective series of blunt and penetrating trauma patients suspected of having sustained cardiac trauma evaluated by 2-D echo gave further credence to the utility of this method in detecting pericardial effusions (Reid et al. 1987).[1] The seminal, prospective study by Jimenez et al. gave rise to additional reports detailing the use of 2-D echo for cardiac trauma, including a 1995 study from the same institution involving 121 patients (Nagy et al. 1995).[2] As the use of 2-D echo increased during the 1990s, stimulated by this paper and supported by a high degree of accuracy, the routine use of diagnostic pericardial window decreased. The use of pericardial examination was incorporated into the focused assessment with sonography for trauma (FAST) in the late 1990s and has remained an important adjunct in the evaluation of penetrating trauma to the chest ever since.

Finally, as experience accumulated with the use of 2-D echo, it was recognized that occasionally cardiac lacerations may decompress into the adjacent pleural space without the accumulation of any significant pericardial blood. Many centers continue to utilize pericardial window in such cases.

REFERENCES

1. Reid CL, Kawanishi DT, Rahimtoola SH, Chandraratna PA. Chest trauma: evaluation by two-dimensional echocardiography. *Am Heart J*. 1987; 113(4): 971–976.
2. Nagy KK, Lohmann C, Kim DO, Barrett J. Role of echocardiography in the diagnosis of occult penetrating cardiac injury. *J Trauma*. 1995; 38(6): 859–862.

Editor Notes: This was one of the first publications to suggest that 2-D echocardiography could replace subziphoid pericardiotomy, or "window," in excluding cardiac injury. Seventy-three patients with chest wounds underwent echo followed by a pericardial window, and 9 of 10 cardiac injuries were identified (96% accuracy). The study led to the routine use of cardiac echo to exclude cardiac injury after penetrating injury in the "zone of death" for individuals without hemothorax.

Limitations:

Small population studies;
Cardiology fellow performed 2-D echo studies;
Unclear if any patients had a hemothorax.

CHAPTER 22

Noninvasive Vascular Tests Reliably Exclude Occult Arterial Trauma in Injured Extremities

Johansen K, Lynch K, Paun M, Copass M. J Trauma
31:515–519; discussion 519–522, 1991

Abstract   We evaluated the ability of noninvasive vascular tests to exclude clinically significant occult arterial damage in injured extremities. In a preliminary study, a Doppler arterial pressure index (API) (the systolic AP in the injured extremity divided by the AP in an uninvolved arm) of less than 0.90 was found to have a sensitivity and specificity of 95% and 97%, respectively, for major arterial injury. The negative predictive value for an API greater than 0.90 was 99%. Because these values suggested that noninvasive vascular tests might effectively be substituted for "exclusion" arteriography in patients at risk for silent extremity arterial injuries, we then conducted a trial in which arteriography was performed in extremity trauma victims only when the API was less than 0.90. Among 100 traumatized limbs (84 penetrating, 16 blunt) in 96 consecutive patients, 16 of 17 limbs (94%) with an API less than 0.90 had positive arteriographic findings, and seven underwent arterial reconstruction. Among 83 limbs with an API greater than 0.90, a follow-up (including duplex scanning in 64 limbs) revealed five minor arterial lesions (four pseudoaneurysms, one arteriovenous fistula) but no major injuries. Arteriograms for extremity trauma fell from 14% to 5.2% of all angiographic studies performed (p less than 0.001, Chi-square). These studies suggest that noninvasive vascular tests can reliably exclude major occult arterial damage in injured extremities. Screening for such injuries with Doppler arterial pressure measurements, reserving arteriography for limbs in which the API is less than 0.90, is safe, accurate, and cost effective.

Author Commentary by Kaj Johansen

Vascular ultrasound originated in the 1960s and 1970s in Seattle via the work of Rushmer, Strandness, and Spencer. Coincidentally, I initiated my academic vascular surgical career at Harborview Medical Center in Seattle at the very time that the clinical applications of Doppler pressure measurements and arterial duplex were being explored (predominantly in patients with chronic arterial occlusive disease). It seemed to me timely to utilize this novel noninvasive tool in various emergency settings; in this case, for the evaluation of patients potentially harboring post-traumatic arterial injuries.

First we showed, in an arteriography-controlled trial of 100 injured extremities in 93 patients, that Doppler-derived ankle-brachial pressure indices (APIs) are highly sensitive and specific for significant extremity arterial injury: positive and negative predictive values for an API = 0.90 were 95% and 97%.[1] Armed with these data, in a subsequent series of 96 patients with 100 injured extremities, we restricted the use of arteriography to patients with an API less than 0.90. In that study, we detected all major arterial injuries, missing only a few minor or inconsequential injuries (pseudoaneurysms, small intimal flaps, AV fistulas). Compared to "traditional" diagnostic protocols of the time we reduced the use of contrast arteriograms in this patient population by 75%.[2]

Shortcomings of this noninvasive approach include the fact that it is useful only in the extremities, fails to detect injuries to non-axial branches, such as the profunda femoris or profunda brachii arteries, and is insensitive to the presence of non-pressure-reducing arterial lesions. Several of these shortcomings were addressed in companion efforts to exploit duplex scanning in the trauma setting.[3]

Others had intimated the potential of such noninvasive techniques in this setting, including Hobson and colleagues in Newark[4] and the LA County-USC group,[5] whose use of a Doppler-derived API threshold of 1.00 proved slightly more sensitive for the detection of occult extremity injuries at the expense of substantially more non-revealing arteriograms performed.

Ultimately the widespread use of whole-body CT scanning in polytrauma victims has mostly supplanted noninvasive arterial assessment as a screening test for occult extremity arterial injuries in most trauma centers. Because such vascular laboratory studies are noninvasive, portable, inexpensive, accurate, and readily repeated, they will likely continue to have value in certain specialized scenarios; for example, in a mass casualty situation when patient assessment is needed immediately, and the CT scanner is not available, or in a rural or developing country setting.

REFERENCES

1. Lynch M, Johansen KH. Can Doppler pressure measurement replace "exclusion" arteriography in extremity trauma? *Ann Surg.* 1991; 214: 737–741.
2. Johansen K, Lynch M, Paun M, Copass M. Non-invasive vascular tests reliably exclude occult arterial injury in extremity trauma. *J Trauma.* 1991; 31: 515–522.
3. Meissner M, Paun M, Johansen K. Duplex scanning for arterial trauma. *Am J Surg.* 1991; 161: 552–555.
4. Anderson RJ, Hobson RW 2nd, Lee BC, et al. Reduced dependency on arteriography for penetrating arterial trauma: Influence of wound location and noninvasive vascular tests. *J Trauma.* 1990; 30: 1059–1063.
5. Schwartz MR, Weaver FA, Bauer M, et al. Refining the indications for arteriography in penetrating extremity trauma: A prospective analysis. *J Vasc Surg.* 1993; 17: 116–122.

Expert Commentary by William Schecter

The modern era of vascular trauma arguably began when Frank Spenser reconstructed an injured femoral artery in 1952 during the Korean War. The epidemic of violence associated with drug use during the 1960s as well as the Vietnam War led to increasing experience with vascular injuries. At that time, surgeons performed single shot angiography in the emergency department or operating room, and this was used to provide a "road map" for selected patients. Mandatory exploration of major vessels in proximity to penetrating injury was widely practiced due to concern for blast injury, pseudoaneurysms, intimal flaps, or arteriovenous fistula.

By the late 1960s, more sophisticated angiography performed in the radiology department became widely available. This procedure rapidly replaced mandatory exploration for proximity as a means to exclude major vascular injury. However, most of the arteriograms were normal. Moreover, increasing experience indicated that most small intimal flaps and arteriovenous fistulas healed spontaneously without surgery.

Many surgeons questioned the value of routine arteriography for the indication of proximity, but Kaj Johansen was the first to apply the arterial pressure index (API) to the assessment of penetrating extremity injuries. This technique, first developed for the evaluation of chronic limb ischemia, proved to be a useful tool for screening patients for angiography. Johansen's careful study tested his hypothesis and proved that the API was an accurate test. This paper led to a decrease in unnecessary diagnostic angiography nationwide.

Johansen hints at the role of Duplex ultrasonography as a noninvasive means of trauma vascular imaging. This technology, available at the time, subsequently improved and found a useful role limited by operator dependency in image interpretation.

The sometimes competing, sometimes complementary techniques of API, Duplex ultrasonography, and interventional arteriography were the tools available in the 1990s. By the turn of the century, two revolutionary technologies appeared: high-resolution computed tomography (CT) and catheter-based endovascular surgery. Now noninvasive CT angiography could rapidly provide spectacular images of vascular injuries, which could easily be seen even by neophyte clinicians. The widespread use of CT in trauma patient evaluation meant that these angiograms were available for most patients.

Endovascular surgery, including the deployment of stents to treat both aneurysmal and occlusive disease, was rapidly applied to the field of vascular trauma. Now interventional angiography regained its prominence, not for diagnosis but for treatment. The story is still unfolding, but there is no doubt that the seminal contribution of Johansen and his colleagues led to a sea change in the vascular evaluation of extremity injuries.

Editor Notes: This paper was a large prospective validation study concerning the accuracy of noninvasive Doppler arterial pressure index (API) to identify injuries in 100 extremities. Patients with "hard" signs of vascular injury were excluded, and those with an API < 0.90 underwent contrast arteriography. Those with API > 0.90 underwent serial examination and duplex sonography. API was highly sensitive and specific for major arterial injury. Prior to this publication, angiography was routinely used for evaluation of patients with "proximity" extremity wounds. This landmark paper challenged the dogma of the day and lead to selective use of angiography in extremity wounds.

Limitations:

Observational trial in just 96 patients with 100 extremity injuries;
Few blunt vascular injuries;
Technique misses some lesions (AV fistula and pseudoaneurysm) and was abnormal in arterial spasm;
Young population studied so not validated in the elderly injured with possibly existing peripheral vascular disease;
And variability in frequency and length of follow-up.

CHAPTER 23

Evaluation of the Necessity of Clinical Observation of High-Energy Trauma Patients without Significant Injury after Standardized Emergency Room Stabilization

Lansink KW, Cornejo CJ, Boeije T, Kok MF, Jurkovich GJ, Ponsen KJ. J Trauma 57(6):1256–1259, 2004

Abstract   This manuscript challenged a widely adopted practice of empiric 24-hour observation of high-energy trauma patients who have no major injuries identified. The underpinning of the paper is the assumption that the initial trauma evaluation is inadequate to identify clinically significant injuries, and that patients would develop new complaints and additional diagnoses during a subsequent in-hospital observation period.

Background   Patients involved in a high-energy trauma (HET) are usually admitted for clinical observation, even when no significant injury is found after standard care in the emergency room (ER). The necessity of this observation period is not evidence based. The goal of this study was to identify patients who revealed an initially undiagnosed injury during the observation period.

Methods   A retrospective study of consecutive HET patients was conducted in two level I trauma centers. Patients after a HET with two minor injuries or less, diagnosed during the standard ER care, were included. Data were abstracted from patients' medical records.

Results   Five hundred three patients were included. None of the patients developed any complications during the clinical observation period or were readmitted to their own hospital within a week after the trauma.

Conclusion   There is no evidence for the necessity of clinical observation of HET patients with minimal or no injuries diagnosed after standard ER stabilization and evaluation.

Expert Commentary by David R. King

The study is a retrospective review conducted at two level I trauma centers (one within the United States and one from the Netherlands) of 503 patients admitted for empiric observation with two or fewer minor injuries identified during their initial trauma evaluation. High-energy trauma was defined using surrogates of high instantaneous change in velocity (e.g., motor vehicle crash with significant passenger compartment intrusion). During the 24-hour observation period, not a single patient developed a complication of late manifestation of an injury. None of the patients were readmitted within 30 days of discharge.

This study reinforced the necessity of surgical scientists to continue to question all practice patterns not solidly based in science. Often, current medical practice masquerades as evidence-based medicine, as was the case when this paper was written. This paper demonstrated that an observation period is not necessary following high-energy trauma with minimal or no injuries, provided that the initial trauma evaluation is detailed and appropriate. Furthermore, these results are generalizable to trauma care in the United States as well as Europe. Interestingly, a minority of patients received axial imaging, a lesson we should remind ourselves of today, more than a decade later.

Expert Commentary by Matthew O. Dolich

Physicians caring for trauma patients perpetually exist between a rock and a hard place—the boundaries of which are fundamentally defined by the entities of overtriage and undertriage. The downside of undertriage is obvious; having a trauma-related preventable death due to treatment at a non-trauma center is clearly an undesirable outcome. The fear of undertriage, and associated litigation, has resulted in an acceptance of relatively high rates of trauma center overtriage, in an attempt to minimize the likelihood of a significant missed injury. However, overtriage has numerous downsides, as well, including hospital-acquired infection, venous thromboembolism, patient dissatisfaction, physician burnout, issues with resident work hour compliance, and education/service balance. Lastly, rising costs associated with inpatient hospitalization is a very real consideration when discussing the impact of overtriage in trauma systems.

Historically, virtually all patients brought to a trauma center after high-energy trauma, such as motor vehicle collisions, were admitted for a period of observation—typically 24 hours. As the authors of this important paper note, "The purpose of this observation period is to detect any late manifestations of a serious or life-threatening injury." However, there are no compelling data supporting a link between the rotational interval of the Earth on its axis and a reduction in missed injury rates. Rather, this practice originated in a different time and has been adhered to, dogmatically, ever since. In many ways, we as trauma surgeons have been slow to realize that an unnecessary overnight stay in the hospital is more than a minor inconvenience. A paradigm shift away from "routine" hospitalization began decades ago in many other specialties. In the 1980s and early 1990s, many low-risk patients with community-acquired pneumonia spent multiple days in the hospital for intravenous antibiotics, close observation, and monitoring of daily chest X-rays. Now, the vast majority of these patients are treated on an outpatient basis, with equivalent or better outcomes. Venous thromboembolism, previously always treated by initial inpatient hospitalization, has followed the same pathway in low-risk patient populations. Similarly, when I began my surgical training in the early 1990s, the common practice for patients undergoing elective colon resection was for admission the day prior to surgery for bowel preparation and IV hydration. The prevailing belief, at the time, was that this preoperative hospitalization would minimize complications related to dehydration and improve outcome after surgery. Now, in the face of evidence to the contrary and negative financial pressure from medical insurance carriers, this practice has been abandoned.

This paper provided crucial early evidence to boost confidence in discharging minimally injured patients directly from the emergency department, despite the high-energy mechanism of injury. Indeed, with hospital costs now estimated at over $2,200 per inpatient day in the United States, minimizing unnecessary hospitalization of overtriaged patients arriving at trauma centers is clearly a goal worth pursuing. By sending uninjured patients home, trauma centers can substantially mitigate unnecessary costs in already overburdened health care system. I now tell my patients that they're going to be happier sleeping in their own beds; they rarely disagree.

Editor Notes: Investigators at two trauma centers assessed the value of hospital admission for exclusion of injuries after negative imaging work-up in patients experiencing high-energy trauma. None of 503 patients developed a complication or was diagnosed with a major missed injury during overnight admission or 30-day follow-up period, thereby proving that admission for clinical observation, after a negative emergency center work-up was unnecessary.

Limitations:

Retrospective review so it is possible that the study missed injuries found subsequently;
Radiation impact not really addressed here, which would be of interest, particularly in children.

CHAPTER 24

Fluid and Electrolyte Requirements in Severe Burns

Evans EI, Purnell OJ, Robinett PW, Batchelor A, Martin M.
Ann Surg 135(6):804–815, 1952

Abstract "Fluid and Electrolyte Requirements in Severe Burns" published by Evans et al. in *Annals of Surgery* in 1952 is a seminal paper in the history of burn care, and the results and conclusions therein provided a giant leap forward in the clinical management of burn-injured patients. The principle finding in this publication, as recognized by the primary reviewer, Dr. Michael DeBakey, was the development of a "simple and practical formula for the calculation of the fluid requirements of the severely burned patient, particularly during the early shock period."

Expert Commentary by Basil A. Pruitt

The authors recorded their experience in the management of 68 burn patients and provided data used for the development of "a simple formula for the calculation of colloid and electrolyte requirements in the extensively burned patient in the first 48 hours." The authors described their early experience illustrating the risk of pulmonary edema associated with the use of a formula based on surface area of the burn alone without consideration of the patient's weight to calculate resuscitation fluid needs in burn patients with inhalation injury, babies and children, patients of ≥50 years, and those with burns of ≥50% of the total body surface area (TBSA).

The evolution of this group's fluid resuscitation regimen, into what came to be known as the "Evans Formula," illustrates the strength of a program of integrated clinical and laboratory research in resolving clinical problems. To address the problem of fluid overload with resuscitation, the authors reduced the calculated volume of colloid fluid to the level of plasma loss per kilogram body weight per % burn observed 24 hours after injury (1.0cc) in the canine burn model they had developed. They arbitrarily added a similar volume of electrolyte containing fluid (1.0 cc/%burn/Kg) noting that, when large salt doses were required, one-third should be a Lactated Ringers solution and two-thirds normal saline. They recommended reduction of both colloid and electrolyte infusion by 50% for the second 24 hours and noted the importance of markedly reducing salt intake from their measured infusion of 90 grams of sodium chloride in the first 48 hours to 4–6 grams daily, thereafter. The authors also emphasized prompt initiation of resuscitation noting that, when resuscitation was delayed, "vigorous" shock therapy was often required with the infused volumes increasing as the delay increased and might, when delay was prolonged, exceed the calculated requirements. Equally important, the authors established a urinary output of 25–50 cc per hour as a range that enabled them to protect both the lung and the kidney from iatrogenic excess or deficit.

The authors included four brief case reports to illustrate their management program for extensively burned patients and document the broad applicability and effectiveness of the Evans Formula. On the basis of this paper and related publications of Dr. Evans, the Evans Formula became a widely used method of estimating early post-burn resuscitation fluid needs. It was used at the US Army Burn Center until Drs. Artz and Reiss reviewed and comparted the resuscitation fluid received by their patients who had lived or died. They found that the survivors had received more electrolyte solution than colloid solution and formulated the Brooke Formula, a lineal descendant of the Evans Formula, which altered the colloid and electrolyte content from 1:1 to 0.5:1.5, respectively. The modified Brooke Formula, a second-generation descendant of the Evans Formula, removed the colloid content in the first 24 hours and increased the electrolyte component to 2.0 mL/%TBSA/Kg. The authors' endorsement of whole blood as the favored fluid for the IV treatment of shock in burn patients has been displaced by the current use of plasma or albumin solutions. The surface area limitation of 50% TBSA for calculating fluid needs has also given way to the use of the total area burned.

The authors recognized that the formulas they proposed should be employed only as a guide to treatment with the actual fluids infused varied according to the patients' response to the injury, and the treatment as assessed hourly. In short, the information in this paper simplified and refined the initial fluid resuscitation of burn patients and has served as the progenitor of current formulae used to predict the resuscitation fluid requirements of burn patients.

Expert Commentary by Kevin N. Foster

At the time of publication of this manuscript, burn care was in its infancy and the mortality from a relatively small burn remained very high. As the authors note in their Introduction, it had been recently recognized that early burn mortality secondary to burn shock was due to loss of fluid from the intravascular space into the periphery. Treatment of this fluid loss and burn shock consisted of fluid infusion adequate to maintain and/or restore perfusion to organs and tissues. However, how much fluid and what type of fluid (colloid or crystalloid) to be used remained to be defined.

This formula for fluid resuscitation was prescient in several ways. First, it utilized the patient's weight and the percent total body surface area (% TBSA) burned as the primary input factors. Second, it utilized the resuscitation fluids consisting of a combination of crystalloid (normal saline and D5W) and colloid (whole blood, plasma, and/or plasma substitutes). Finally, monitoring the effectiveness of resuscitation was maintenance of urine output between 25 and 50 cc per hour. With the exception of the use of whole blood, this paradigm is very similar to the resuscitation protocols used by most modern burn centers.

This manuscript also presented several other findings that remain applicable to burn care. Because the resuscitation formula requires the determination of % TBSA burned, the authors presented an easy and accurate method for estimating the extent of burn injury by dividing the body into areas of 9% and 18% TBSA. This is known as the Rule of Nines and is still widely used to quickly estimate the extent of burn injury.

The authors also report the Rule of 50, emphasizing the difficulties associated with resuscitating older patients (>age 50) and patients with large %TBSA burns (>50% TBSA). This remains true today although most burn care providers would cite a rule of 70 or 80. Similarly, the authors also report that patients with burns of less than 20%–25% TBSA likely do not require formal fluid resuscitation, which is the current standard of care.

Finally, the authors also presaged the development of "fluid creep" or over-resuscitation with the report of patients who developed pulmonary edema and had high mortality because of aggressive fluid infusions.

An interesting point made in the Introduction was the importance of developing an effective burn resuscitation formula because of the fear of thousands of burn victims due to atomic warfare. This paper was published during the early Cold War years.

Editor Notes: This was one of the first studies to resuscitate severe burn victims using a fixed-fluid protocol (colloid plus crystalloid) during the first 24 hours of admission. The monitoring of urine output was stressed, as well as the use of whole blood for the management of "burn shock." In 1951, they found that up to 20% body surface area burns did universally well, while burns of greater than 40% were often fatal.

Limitations:

Observational descriptive study;
Small patient population studied (n = 68);
Fixed formula does not account for depth of the burn, 0.75 cc colloid (plasma)
plus 0.75 cc crystalloid solutions were given for each percent body surface area
of burn for the first 24 hours of hospitalization.

CHAPTER 25

The Diagnosis of the Depth of Burning

Jackson DM. Br J Surg 40(164):588–596, 1953

Abstract   The relevance of this monograph lies in its meticulous description of the temporal evolution of burned skin in the first 3 weeks. Using the most recent classification of burns based on depth of tissue destruction (not outward appearance), that being partial and full-thickness, Jackson outlines the clinical and histological appearances of burned skin seen over this time. His classification of the intensity of burning of the dermis, or the three zones of injury, provided the groundwork for our current understanding of the pathophysiology of thermal injury to the skin.

Expert Commentary by Christopher E. White

Surgical principles dictate early excision of devitalized tissue and prompt wound closure for all traumatic wounds. In this article, published in 1953, Dr. Jackson, MD, FRCS, underscores this argument for the rapid identification and closure of full-thickness burn wounds. For 20–30 years prior to this publication, small, well-defined burns of 2%–3% total body surface area (TBSA) were completely excised and grafted with good results.[1] Although successful, the experience in the mid-1950s with early excision and grafting of burns of 10%–30% TBSA and larger showed the overall mortality and wound healing were not different from delayed treatment, which consisted of allowing the burn eschar to separate from underlying granulation tissue followed by delayed grafting.[2,3] Early excision and grafting, however, was largely the accepted method for very deep burns of <20% TBSA since it may take 6 weeks or more for the eschar to slough and separate.[4] Graft failure, in these cases, was partly attributed to infection of the surrounding unexcised burn. Additionally, it wasn't until the next decade that the development of topical agents such as 0.5% $AgNO_3$, 1% Silversulfadiazine, and 10% Sulfamylon ointments were shown to provide significant suppression of burn wound sepsis.[5]

During the first day after injury, the burn may be described by three zones: the zone of hyperemia (peripheral), the zone of stasis (intermediate), and the zone of coagulation (central) (Figure 25.1). The outer zone remains perfused and blanches with pressure. Histological section shows near complete loss of the epidermis without damage to the dermis; consequently, the outer zone should heal spontaneously. The central zone of coagulation received the maximal damage resulting in cell death and will require debridement. On light microscopy, it is characterized by complete obliteration of the lumina of the vessels in the

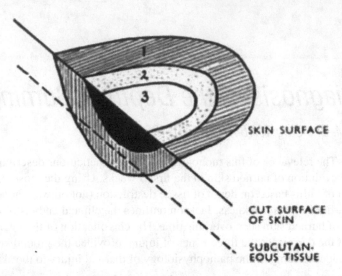

Figure 25.1   Shows the three zones of intensity: (1) The zone of hyperaemia (peripheral). (2) The zone of stasis (intermediate). (3) The zone of coagulation (central). (*Source:* Jackson, DM. The diagnosis of the depth of burning. *Br J Surg.* 1953; 40: 588–596.)

subpapillary plexus and capillary loops. The intermediate zone is characterized by decreased tissue perfusion and metabolism, and although viable early, it may progress to coagulation necrosis with additional insults, such as hypotension, infection, or continued inflammation and edema. Coagulated or necrotic cells, in addition to being a nidus for infection, are a source of inflammatory mediators, which may cause capillary leakage, edema, hypercoagulabilty, and thrombosis in the intermediate zone promoting further ischemia and cell death.[6] In fact, Jackson reported white mottling of the zone of stasis between the third and seventh day so that only the hyperemic outer and the white central zones were then present. Maintenance of good wound perfusion, especially during burn shock, and the early excision and immediate grafting of dead tissue may spare the intermediate zone of full-thickness conversion.

REFERENCES

1. Ross WPD. The treatment of recent burns of the hand. *Br J Plast Surg.* 1950; 2: 233.
2. MacMillan BG. Early excision of more than twenty-five percent of body surface in the extensively burned patient; an evaluation. *Arch Surg.* 1958; 77: 369.
3. Jackson DM, Topley E, Cason JS, Lowbury EJL. Primary excision and grafting of large burns. *Ann Surg.* 1960; 152: 167.
4. Jackson DM. *Proc Roy Soc Med.* 1971; 65: 23–24.
5. Quinby WC, Burke JF, Bondoc CC. Primary excision and immediate wound closure. *Int Care Med.* 1981; 7: 71–76.
6. Salibian AA, Rosario ATD, Severo LAM, et al. Current concepts on burn wound conversion: A review of recent advances in understanding the secondary progressions of burns. *Burns.* 2016; 42: 1025–1035.

Editor Notes: One of the first reports to describe the concept of partial-thickness and full-thickness burns delineated the zones of hyperemia, stasis, and coagulation, and how the burn pathology progressed over the first few weeks.

Limitations:

Observational descriptive study;
No validation analysis relating depth of burns with patient outcomes;
Little data included.

CHAPTER 26

Management of the Major Coagulopathy with Onset during Laparotomy

Stone HH, Strom PR, Mullins RJ. Ann Surg 197(5):532–535, 1983

Abstract   An experience with 31 patients who developed major bleeding diatheses during laparotomy was reviewed. Management of the initial 14 patients was by standard hematologic replacement, completion of all facets of operation, and then closure of the peritoneal cavity, usually with suction drainage; only one patient survived. The subsequent 17 patients had laparotomy terminated as rapidly as possible to avoid additional bleeding. Major vessel injuries were repaired; ends of resected bowel were ligated; and holes in other gastrointestinal segments and the bladder were closed by purse-string sutures. One patient had a ureter ligated. Laparotomy pads (4–17) were then packed within the abdomen to effect tamponade, and the abdomen was closed under tension without drains or stomata. Following correction of the coagulopathy, the abdomen was re-explored at 15–69 hours in the 12 survivors. Definitive surgery then was completed: bowel resection and reanastomosis; ureter reimplantation; drains for bile, pancreatic juice, and urine; and stomata for bowel or urine diversion or decompression. Eleven of 17 patients, deemed to have a lethal coagulopathy, survived. This technique of initial abortion of laparotomy, establishment of intra-abdominal pack tamponade, and then completion of the surgical procedure once coagulation has returned to an acceptable level has proven to be lifesaving in previously non-salvageable situations.

Author Commentary by H. Harlan Stone

The following was compiled from Dr. Stone's[1] written commentary and an interview with him on June 7, 2018.

> The techniques described in the article in question, resulted from my experience at the Grady Hospital. We didn't have any attendings ever! I just took call every night, from home. I was probably scrubbed every other night. I had control of 140 beds. It was the experience treating patients with necrotizing pancreatitis, my pediatric surgical experience treating omphalocele, and the treatment of patients with injury to large vascular structures and a coagulopathy that led us to treat patients in this manner.

As detailed in the article cited for this discussion,[1] perhaps the most disastrous situation faced by the trauma surgeon is an open abdomen in the patient whose blood will not clot.

Immediately on noting coagulopathy (i.e., absence of fresh clots), the abdomen was closed tightly. The laws of hydrodynamics are to be honored: flow occurs only when pressure in the feeding reservoir sufficiently exceeds that of the receiving basin. Application of this principle was clearly shown by Richards et al. in 1966.[2] Only arterial bleeders are to be addressed by repair of ligature before abdominal closure. This significantly increased intra-abdominal pressure will arrest all but a trickle of blood.

Quickly the abdominal cavity was packed with sutured lap pads (or preferably sterile cotton hand towels or small bath towels obtained from a local Walmart). The sub-diaphragmatic gutters were first packed laterally for medial compression of liver fracture lines between lobes, segments, and sub-segments. This is where torn hepatic veins are located in cases of blunt trauma. Next, the pelvis was packed, followed by extra pads or towels to sufficiently fill the abdominal cavity. No time was taken to close bowel holes or organ resection, except for an injured spleen. A large running monofilament suture was used to approximate under tension the incision walls. If massive bowel edema precluded one's ability to close fascia, then the skin alone was sewn with a baseball type of stitch. We left no drains or stomas, for they would have allowed a seepage that prevented the creation of the needed compartment pressure.

Now an abdominal compartment syndrome must be managed. This is exactly what surgeons faced in the early 1900s when correcting large omphaloceles (i.e., gaps greater than 5 cm) in newborns. If clearly too tight, the infant would first have tachycardia, followed by bradycardia, and then death. The significantly increased intra-abdominal pressure would have compressed the cava and other veins so as to prevent adequate return of blood to the heart from the abdomen and lower torso. Fascial closure would then immediately be abandoned and then a ventral hernia created with only skin approximation. In 6 weeks to 6 months, this midline hernia would be corrected.

Upon re-entry into the trauma patient's peritoneal cavity, all packing was removed and counted. Only then were the needed repair procedures done. However, the first item was a renal decapsulation.[3] Only one kidney was done; the left was more easily exposed. Care was taken to strip the capsule alone, never the cortex. Benefit was readily seen in a postoperative comparative renal scan. There then followed routine correction of all other visceral injuries.

Considerable bowel edema usually prevented a fascial closure, so once again reliance on the ventral hernia was chosen. Just as with infants, hernia repair was delayed for 6 weeks to 6 months.

Critical to all of the above described management is the cool head of a knowledgeable and intelligent surgeon. For those there can be no substitute.

REFERENCES

1. Stone HH, Strom DR, Mullins RJ. Management of the major coagulopathy with onset during laparotomy. *Ann Surg.* 1983; 197: 532–535.
2. Richards AJ Jr., Lamis PA Jr., Rogers JP Jr., Bradham GB. Laceration of abdominal aorta and study of intact abdominal wall as taponade; report of survival and literature review. *Ann Surg.* 1966; 164: 321–324.
3. Stone HH, Fulenwider JT. Renal decapsulation in the prevention of post-ischemic oliguria. *Ann Surg.* 1977; 186: 343–355.

Expert Commentary by Michael F. Rotondo

I vividly recall reading this paper in 1991 and saying to myself, "This is it—this is the answer." I discovered this manuscript, written nearly a decade earlier, in the *Annals of Surgery* via an old fashioned, before-the-Internet-style literature search: look for a decent current paper on the topic of interest, and pull all the references from that paper and from all the references of references until you had all the relevant information. And in that process of digging and sifting for how to approach penetrating injury patients with overwhelming abdominal exsanguination, there it was.

At that time, during the early years of the development of the Trauma Center at University of Pennsylvania, we were encountering patients who defied most of the available literature on penetrating injury. With the change in wounding mechanisms due to ready access of higher caliber, rapid firing semi-automatic weaponry, we were seeing patients with multiple penetrations, massive haemorrhage, and rapidly devolving physiology—cold, acidotic, coagulopathic—patients who were well on the way to dying. While luminaries in the field, like Lucas, Legerwood, and Feliciano, had suggested that the use of temporizing laparotomy had utility for blunt injuries to the liver—few if any had suggested that temporizing laparotomy may have a role in penetrating injury.

As evidenced by this landmark work, Dr. Stone, by the early 1980s, had reached the conclusion that patients who become coagulopathic during exploration for penetrating injury simply die—there must be another way. In a simple report on 17 patients who "were deemed to have lethal coagulopathy," 11 of 17 survived after initial "aborted laparotomy"—"repair of only those vessels to survive"—"ligation of bowel ends" and "abdominal tamponade" with packing. There it was, the answer.

This seminal work formed the foundation of our research and clinical work at Penn in the 1990s and led us to describe the three-stage concept of Damage Control Surgery:

1. Initial control of hemorrhage and contamination, intra-abdominal packing, and temporary abdominal closure;

2. Restoration of normal physiology;
3. Definitive laparotomy with reconstruction.

If you comb carefully through Dr. Stone's manuscript, you will find it all: details on the conduct of the first operation—tips on managing vascular injuries, solid organs and hollow viscera—the utility of closing only the skin—the need for ICU vigilance, hemodynamic support, and blood product administration—high pressure ventilator support and the problems of increased intra-abdominal pressure—and, of course, full details on the conduct of the secondary operation. It's all there. Were it not for this paper, heavily referenced around the country by those interested in these challenging patients, the concept of Damage Control Surgery, popularized more than a decade after this publication, may never have come to fruition. And were it not for the widespread use of Damage Control Surgery during the wars in Iraq and Afghanistan, perhaps the concept of Damage Control Resuscitation may not have come to fruition either. Evidence that this work has been and will be enduring for years to come.

Editor Notes: This was one of the first papers to suggest improved outcomes in patients with coagulopathy and bleeding by terminating abdominal surgery in unstable patients. Almost universal mortality was described in a historical control group when abdominal operations were continued until completion (13/14 died), as compared to 6/17 deaths when a protocol of early packing and abbreviated laparotomy and return to the operating room after restoration of normal physiologic parameters was employed. Today, patients with hemodynamic instability, worsening acidosis, hypothermia, and coagulopathy undergo early termination of their procedures with planned returns to the operating theater.

Limitations:

Retrospective review of data using historical controls;
Limited data on the groups being compared.

CHAPTER 27

Mortality in Retroperitoneal Hematoma

Selivanov V, Chi HS, Alverdy JC, Morris JA Jr,
Sheldon GF. J Trauma 24(12):1022–1027, 1984

Abstract   Eighty-one patients sustained retroperitoneal hematoma (RH) from blunt (70%) and penetrating (30%) trauma. Retroperitoneal hematomas were classified into 10 centro-medial Zone I, 25 lateral Zone II, and 46 pelvic Zone III hematomas. The mean Injury Severity Score (ISS) for the entire series was 26.4 ± 14. The mean ISS of nonsurvivors was 37.6 ± 12. Overall mortality was 20%; if head injury deaths are excluded (six), mortality was 13%. Retroperitoneal hematoma associated with pelvic fracture had a mortality of 19%. Incidence of respiratory failure for entire series, excluding head trauma, was 29%. Respiratory failure occurred in 37% of patients with Zone III injuries. A requirement for ventilatory support greater than 48 hours was associated with a mortality of 35%. PaO_2/FIO_2 at 48 hours in intubated patients was significantly decreased in nonsurvivors compared to survivors, whereas the mean ISS of this subset of patients did not differentiate between survivors and nonsurvivors.

Author Commentary by John A. Morris

Overview   This paper by Selivanov and Sheldon was written in the early 1980s, at an inflection point in the diagnosis of traumatic intra-abdominal hemorrhage. Historically, the need for trauma laparotomy was defined by physical examination, followed by diagnostic peritoneal lavage and, finally, high-resolution CT scan and ultrasound. Each of these modalities had a high false-positive rate: 30% for physical examination, 10%–12% for DPL, but less than 1% for CT scan.[1,2] In the 1980s, unsuspected retroperitoneal hematoma (RH) was found at laparotomy in both blunt (70% of RH) and penetrating (30% of RH) patients.[3,4] The mortality rate of RH, at that time, varied between 18% and 31%.[3,5–7]

In the early 1980s, three classification schemes for RH were advanced.[4,8–10] Each attempted to provide guidelines for intraoperative exploration of the hematoma. All were based on anatomy (zone of injury) and mechanism of injury (blunt versus penetrating).

Sheldon's guidelines, created in 1982, had the widest acceptance because of their simplicity. Intraoperatively, all centro-medial (Zone I) hematomas were explored. Flank hematomas (Zone II) were explored if IVP revealed a renal injury requiring repair, or if the hematoma was expanding. Zone III hematomas, due to pelvic injuries, were not explored unless the hematoma was rapidly expanding.[8]

In the late 1980s, Feliciano proposed a useful modification to Sheldon's scheme, delineating the management of midline supra-mesocolic hematomas.[9] Because of the high likelihood of major vascular injury, Feliciano stated that supra-mesocolic hematomas should only be opened after obtaining proximal and distal vascular control.

The Selivanov manuscript attempts to reinforce the Sheldon classification guidelines with outcome data. Eighty-one patients sustained retroperitoneal hematoma from blunt (70% of patients) and penetrating (30% of patients) trauma. Retroperitoneal hematomas were further classified as centro-medial Zone I (10 patients), lateral Zone II (25 patients), and pelvic Zone III (46 patients) hematomas. Thirty-seven percent of patients were hypotensive on admission. Overall mortality (excluding patients with head injury) was 13%. Retroperitoneal hematomas associated with pelvic fractures had a mortality of 19%.[11]

Strengths   The Selivanov manuscript was well received and, virtually, universally adopted by the trauma community. However, less than a year later, Sheldon's group published the first in a long series of papers examining the role of CT scan in blunt abdominal trauma, which would render the scheme proposed by Selivanov obsolete.[12] A review of today's literature reveals virtually no articles on the subject of traumatic RH in the past 10 years, with the exception of registry reviews from developing countries without universal access to CT scan.

Weaknesses   While the Sheldon classification scheme is useful, the manuscript is purely descriptive. The attempt to link the classification scheme to an outcome is challenging. This retrospective analysis, which predates trauma registries, relies on data from a single institution and is underpowered statistically.

While mortality is a legitimate outcome criterion, there is no evidence that the classification scheme had any impact on mortality. Other outcome criteria, such as respiratory failure (patients requiring ventilator support for more than 48 hours), are more likely a function of impaired physiologic reserve (blood loss, resuscitation) rather than a result of the zone of injury.

Current Management   The management of RH has been revolutionized by the widespread introduction of high-resolution CT, the employment of interventional radiology to control hemorrhage, and the widespread use of the ultrasound FAST exam for screening patients. The current management strategy of RH involves identifying a vascular blush on a CT traumagram, and subsequent endovascular embolization by interventional radiology coupled with aggressive resuscitation with blood products.

REFERENCES

1. Federle MP. Computed tomography of blunt abdominal trauma. *Radiol Clin North Am.* 1983; 138: 637–643.
2. Federle MP. CT of abdominal trauma. In: Federle MP, Brant-Zawadzki M, eds. *CT in the Evaluation of Trauma.* Baltimore, MD: Williams & Wilkins; 1982: 71–234.
3. Grieco JG, Perry JF Jr. Retroperitoneal hematoma following trauma: Its clinical significance. *J Trauma.* 1980; 20: 733–736.
4. Henao F, Aldrete JS. Retroperitoneal hematomas of traumatic origin. *Surg Gynecol Obstet.* 1985; 161: 106–116.
5. Allen RE, Eastman BA, Malter BL, et al. Retroperitoneal hemorrhage secondary to blunt trauma. *Am J Surg.* 1969; 118: 588.
6. Baylis SM, Lansing EM, Glas WW. Traumatic retroperitoneal hematoma. *Am J Surg.* 1962; 103: 477–480.
7. Nick WV, Zollinger RW, Pace WG. Retroperitoneal hematoma after blunt abdominal trauma. *J Trauma.* 1967; 7: 652–659.
8. Kudsk KA, Sheldon GF. Retroperitoneal hematoma. In: Blaisdell FW, Trunkey DD, eds. *Abdominal Trauma.* New York: Thieme-Stratton; 1982: 279–293.
9. Feliciano DV, Burch JM, Graham JM. Abdominal vascular injury. In: Mattox KL, Moore EE, Feliciano DV, eds. *Trauma.* East Norwalk, CT: Appleton & Lange; 1988: 519–536.
10. Shafton GW. Retroperitoneal trauma. *Contemp Surg.* 1980; 16: 25–35.
11. Selivanov V, Chi HS, Alverdy JC, et al. Mortality in retroperitoneal hematoma. *J Trauma.* 1984; 24: 1022–1027.
12. Wing VW, Federle MP, Morris JA Jr, et al. The clinical impact of CT for blunt abdominal trauma. *AJR.* 1985; 145: 1191–1194.

Expert Commentary by D. Dante Yeh

"*...expanding Zone I retroperitoneal hematoma...*" Upon reading that short phrase, every trauma surgeon in practice today will likely experience a quickening of the pulse and a tightening of the sphincter. It is without exaggeration that a single "landmark study" can lead an entire community of medical professionals to envision a shared mental model and experience the same visceral response. In one compact monograph, the Selivanov landmark study beautifully illustrates Sheldon's taxonomy, describes its prognostic significance, reports outcome data, and points to areas for future improvement.[1] The Figure 1 schematic that overlays the retroperitoneal zones over a stylized human body is simple, timeless, and not easily forgettable.

Some may view this manuscript, published in 1984, as quaint and outdated. The term "damage control surgery" would not appear until 1993,[2] and pre-peritoneal pelvic packing would not be described until 1995.[3] Resuscitative endovascular balloon occlusion of the aorta (REBOA) would not experience its renaissance for at least another quarter century. However, one can see the seeds of our modern practice germinating from the authors' minds. For example, they report that 9 of the 27 initially stable patients underwent delayed laparotomy for development of hemodynamic instability and they lament that in these 9 patients, "preoperative computed tomography may have allowed avoidance of exploratory laparotomy." This understated comment almost certainly inspired others to revisit the indications for operative exploration in stable (and even unstable) patients. For example, pioneering studies in urologic trauma from the same institution (San Francisco General Hospital) would later report the success of nonoperative management of almost all blunt renal injuries and nearly half of penetrating renal injuries,[4] and other groups would even report the superiority of nonoperative management for *penetrating* renal injury.[5] Endovascular repair is now preferred over open repair for elective and urgent treatment of abdominal aortic degenerative pathology as well as for contained thoracic aortic trauma. Why shouldn't it be the case for Zone I retroperitoneal hematomas encountered in the operating room as well? Indeed, a recent multicenter prospective observational study confirms that endovascular techniques are already being utilized in increasing frequency for non-compressible torso trauma of both blunt and penetrating etiology.[6]

By providing predictive validity evidence and establishing a baseline outcomes assessment for future comparisons, Selivanov's paper codifies the Sheldon taxonomy into the canon of trauma literature and provides the yardstick by which future RH studies are measured. As a fossilized snapshot of trauma practice and outcomes at a time of shifting paradigms and emerging technology, it is fascinating and prophetic. Perhaps one day, technological advances will lead future generations to adopt a "no-zone" approach to the retroperitoneum, as in the fate of the zones of the neck.[7] However, Sheldon's zones of the retroperitoneum will remain a vital part of our oral teaching tradition and the significance of this landmark study will continue unabated.

REFERENCES

1. Selivanov V, et al. Mortality in retroperitoneal hematoma. *J Trauma.* 1984; 24(12): 1022–1027.
2. Rotondo MF, et al. 'Damage control': An approach for improved survival in exsanguinating penetrating abdominal injury. *J Trauma.* 1993; 35(3): 375–382; discussion 382–383.
3. Pohlemann T, Gänsslen A, Bosch U, Tscherne H. The technique of packing for control of hemorrhage in complex pelvic fractures. *Tech Orthop.* 1995; 9(4): 267–270.
4. Meng MV, Brandes SB, McAninch JW. Renal trauma: Indications and techniques for surgical exploration. *World J Urol.* 1999; 17(2): 71–77.
5. Bjurlin MA, et al. Comparison of nonoperative management with renorrhaphy and nephrectomy in penetrating renal injuries. *J Trauma.* 2011; 71(3): 554–558.
6. Faulconer ER, et al. Use of open and endovascular surgical techniques to manage vascular injuries in the trauma setting: A review of the American Association for the Surgery of Trauma PROspective Observational Vascular Injury Trial registry. *J Trauma Acute Care Surg.* 2018; 84(3): 411–417.
7. Shiroff AM, et al. Penetrating neck trauma: A review of management strategies and discussion of the 'No Zone' approach. *Am Surg.* 2013; 79(1): 23–29.

Editor Notes: This paper retrospectively reviewed the location and outcome of 81 trauma victims with retroperitoneal hematomas. This study improved our understanding of the risks of injury to the various zones and helped us categorize hematomas in these areas so that it was possible to devise new management strategies.

Limitations:

Retrospective analysis;
Single center experience with an empiric management protocol;
Limited population size (n = 81 patients);
Injury zones were arbitrarily defined and somewhat overlapping;
CT rarely utilized;
Mortality was mostly related to brain injury among those with multiple blunt trauma (15/16 deaths).

CHAPTER 28

A Technique for the Exposure of the Third and Fourth Portions of the Duodenum

Cattell RB, Braasch JW. Surg Gynecol Obstet 111:378–379, 1960

Expert Commentary by David A. Spain

Cattell and Braasch took advantage of embryology: between the eleventh and thirteenth week of fetal life, the midgut enters the abdominal cavity, turns counterclockwise around the superior mesenteric artery, and then the right colon fuses to the retroperitoneum. By excising this line of fusion and fully mobilizing the mesentery, the Cattell-Brassch maneuver (or by the non-eponymous right medial visceral rotation) allows for full exposure of the duodenum, and the authors note this "has been found useful in dealing with neoplasm, ulceration or perforation occurring in the third and fourth portions of the duodenum."[1]

The first description that I could find in the literature of adopting the Cattell-Braasch maneuver for trauma came from Buscaglia, Blaisdell, and Lim from San Francisco General Hospital in 1969.[2] They reported their approach to 33 patients with various penetrating abdominal vascular injuries. Right medial visceral rotation was their preferred approach for exposure of injuries involving the infrarenal aorta or vena cava. Interestingly, they also describe the technique of left medial visceral rotation, "which is preferred in injury of the suprarenal aorta, left renal artery, superior mesenteric artery, or the celiac axis, the dissection is initiated along the fusion line between the left colon and the lateral posterior peritoneum."[2] In line with the original purpose of this maneuver, in 1979, DeMars et al. first reported using this approach to expose and repair blunt duodenal perforations in 10 patients.[3]

Richard B. Cattell, MD (1900–1964) spent his surgical career at the Lahey Clinic, where he succeeded Dr. Lahey as the clinic director. He was a pioneer in reconstructive biliary surgery and a master thyroid surgeon. John W. Braasch, MD, PhD (1922–2017) also spent his professional career at the Lahey Clinic, where he served as Chair of the Department of Surgery and also founded their general surgery residency program. Over the long term of their combined careers, they were highly regarded for the quality of their patient care, surgical skills, training of surgeons, and numerous contributions to the literature. But this simple piece—not even a case report; one page of text and three drawings with no P-values, propensity matching, or multivariable regression models—a purely descriptive article that described a technique for exposing the third and fourth portion of the duodenum permanently changed the way we expose and control the major infrarenal vasculature.[1]

REFERENCES

1. Cattell RB, Braasch JW. A technique for the exposure of the third and fourth portions of the duodenum. *Surg Gynecol Obstet*. 1960; 111: 378–379.
2. Buscaglia LC, Blaisdell FW, Lim RC Jr. Penetrating abdominal vascular injuries. *Arch Surg*. 1969; 99: 764–769.
3. DeMars JJ, Bubrick MP, Hitchcock CR. Duodenal perforation in blunt abdominal trauma. *Surgery*. 1979; 86: 632–638.

Expert Commentary by Lenworth Jacobs

The paper by Cattell and Braasch addressed an important issue in pancreatico-duodenal surgery. The authors recognized that surgeons were having difficulty in exposing and performing procedures for pancreatic and distal duodenum problems.

They reviewed the embryological development and anatomy of the gastrointestinal tract. They understood that the developmental rotation of the post gastric enteron resulted in the rotation of the small bowel and its mesenteric blood supply, and the ultimate lateral attachment of the right colon to the right paracolic gutter. The procedure they described revolutionized exposure to the third and fourth portions of the duodenum, the inferior vena cava, and the renal vessels.

The simple maneuver of taking down the "white line" and medially rotating the entire right colon, staying in the loose areolar plane, yielded excellent exposure of the inferior vena cava from the bifurcation of the iliac vessels to the inferior border of the liver. It also exposed the renal vessels and the right kidney. It also exposed the plane posterior to the head of the pancreas and allowed for digital dissection of the neck and body of the pancreas. The posterior aspect of the second portion of the duodenum and the inferior aspect of the third and fourth portion of the duodenum were also exposed. This made it easy for pancreatico-duodenal surgical excisions for neoplastic or inflammatory conditions.

This exposure, although originally described for pancreaticoduodenal conditions, has secured a real place in the armamentarium of the trauma surgeon. Injuries to the inferior vena cava either from penetrating causes, such as a knife or a bullet, or from blunt forces that tear the lumbar tributaries off the inferior vena cava, or injuries to the lumbar aorta, result in profuse hemorrhage.

The blood rapidly flows into the loose areolar tissues in the retroperitoneum and into the mesentery and then into the peritoneal cavity.

The surgeon is faced with a massive hemoperitoneum with clots in the peritoneal cavity as well as in the mesentery. It is frequently difficult to identify and pinpoint the exact source of bleeding in the sea of blood, clotted blood, and dissected mesentery. Any vigorous or rough dissection may make the situation worse by enlarging the laceration in the inferior vena cava.

The Cattell-Braasch maneuver is an excellent way to very quickly take down and sweep the right colon medially and place the entire right colon and the appendix along with the right colic artery and the mesenteric vascular arcade up onto the left upper quadrant.

Care must be taken to avoid injuries and disruption of the right testicular vessels from the aorta and the inferior vena cava. Once the posterior retroperitoneum has been widely exposed, it is easy to identify the site and severity of the vascular injury to the inferior vena cava or the renal pedicle vessels. The injury can then be repaired. A more leisurely exploratory laparotomy can be performed while anesthesia is replacing the severe blood loss.

This maneuver is now a formal part of the Advanced Trauma Operative Management (ATOM) course and has saved hundreds of patients with massive exsanguination from the inferior vena cava and other retroperitoneal vessels.

Editor Notes: Cattell describes his procedure for exposure of the duodenum. This technique has been used for decades by general surgeons for expeditious exposure of the right kidney, IVC, duodenum, and head of the pancreas.

Limitations:

No data included, just a technical description.

CHAPTER 29

Management of Perforating Colon Trauma: Randomization between Primary Closure and Exteriorization

Stone HH, Fabian TC. Ann Surg 190(4):430–435, 1979

Abstract   During a 44-month trial, 268 patients with wounds of the colon were entered into a prospective, randomized, nonblinded study. Consideration for primary closure demanded the following: preoperative shock was never profound, blood loss was less than 20% of estimated normal volume, no more than two intra-abdominal organ systems had been injured, fecal contamination was minimal, operation was begun within 8 hours, and wounds of the colon and abdominal wall were never so destructive as to require resection. Once such criteria had been satisfied, colon wound management was dictated by the last digit in the randomly assigned hospital number; odd indicated primary closure; even indicated exteriorization of the wound or primary closure with protection by a proximal vent. Results obtained in 139 determinant patients eligible for randomization revealed that primary closure (67 patients) had a lower infection rate of the incision (48% vs. S7%, p > 0.05) and a still lower infection rate for the abdomen proper (15% vs. 29%, p < 0.05), compared to the 72 patients with a randomized colostomy. Morbidity otherwise for the randomized colostomy was tenfold greater than if a primary closure had been performed. Average postoperative stay was 6 days longer (p < 0.01) if a colostomy had been created, exclusive of subsequent hospitalization for colostomy closure; while the total extra cost for management of the colon wound by colostomy was approximately $2,700.00. Although immediate mortalities were identical, one late death occurred following colostomy closure. These data not only confirm the safety of primary closure for colon wounds in selected cases, but also indicate that such should become the preferred method of treatment whenever specific criteria have been met.

Author Commentary by Timothy C. Fabian

I need to begin by acknowledging that the design and execution of this work was done almost entirely by my mentor Dr. Stone. At the time of publication, I was a trauma fellow with him at Emory University and Grady Memorial Hospital. He was the sole faculty member managing one of the highest volume trauma services in the country, and he most likely had the largest personal experience of any surgeon in the world managing penetrating trauma. He applied that experience well.

Dr. Stone has been one of the most productive clinical investigators in surgery over the past half century. He was one of the first surgeons in the United States who conducted significant numbers of prospective, randomized trials. These led to huge contributions in the management of multiple aspects of trauma and surgical infection.

A backdrop to this particular study is in order. At that time, primary closure of colon wounds was almost strictly verboten. Surgeons were trained to always exteriorize colon injuries as colostomies because of a perceived high risk of suture line failure with primary repair, resulting in high mortality. Historically, exteriorization evolved from surgical care in World War II. It became a uniform practice in British and American armies during the North African Campaign of 1942. When surgeons returned from the war, that practice was perpetuated. Alton Ochsner at Charity Hospital in New Orleans and others began questioning that management around 1960. A few scattered reports of success-ful primary repair surfaced in the 1970s. Our study was designed to objectively address the issue head-on.

A selected group of patients was identified for randomization between primary repair and exteriorization. In an abundance of caution, the most seriously injured patients (shock, blood loss > 1000 mL, major fecal contamination, destructive wounds requiring resection) were not randomized and were managed by the "standard of care." Approximately half of wounds (129) met those severity crite-ria, and the remainder (139) were randomized. Computer randomization was not available at the time (there were no computers!), and so patients were randomized by the traditional Grady approach, by the last digit of their hospital number. Odd numbers resulted in primary repair. Cutting to the chase—primary repair resulted in less intra-abdominal infection and no colon-related deaths. Exteriorizations had 10% ostomy complications, and overall costs were substantially lower with primary repair. The study unequivocally demonstrated that primary repair was superior to the "standard of care" in this selected group of patients. Over the years, other studies reproduced those results and criteria have expanded so that now essentially all nondestructive wounds are managed by primary repair and the majority of destructive wounds are managed by resection and anastomosis. It was an honor to be involved in what I believe was a true landmark study in trauma.

Clinical research methodologies have advanced in leaps and bounds since 1979. We now have computers! Statistical methodologies have become a complex science unto themselves. At the time of this study, Institutional Review Boards (IRBs) were just developing. The National Research Act of 1974 and the Belmont Report of 1979 resulted in widespread IRB development in the early 1980s. Informed consent was not considered at the time of this study. The protection of human subjects has produced a tremendous advance in clinical research. But, research in emergency health care has become complex and difficult. Navigating the waiver of consent process is not for the faint of heart. Nonetheless, prospective, randomized trials remain the *sine qua non* for most medical advances. I encourage young investigators to prepare themselves as clinical trialists by pursuing the advanced education required for this challenging field.

Expert Commentary by Mark A. Malangoni

This report by Harlan Stone and Tim Fabian was a "game changer." They have recounted the background, primarily from military conflicts earlier in the twentieth century, that mandated colostomy or primary repair with exteriorization of the injured area as the only safe treatment of colon injuries. This was challenged by surgeons in the civilian setting, where overall injury burden and colon injury in particular were often less extensive.

The authors prospectively evaluated the outcomes of primary repair of colon injury and exteriorization of the injury either as a colostomy or following repair. The eligibility criteria were stringent, and they excluded patients with coexisting conditions thought to result in a greater likelihood of suture line disruption with primary repair. This study was done over nearly four years and, although prospective, was not randomized or blinded based on today's criteria. Resuscitation, perioperative antimicrobials, and postoperative care were done according to contemporary standards. Nearly half of the patients with colon injury did not meet entry criteria and had mandatory colostomy. Only a single patient died in the study group, and 15% in those who had obligatory colostomy. The infection rate was 15% among patients randomized to primary repair, while those randomized to exteriorization had nearly twice the incidence of infection and had outcomes remarkably similar to the obligatory colostomy patient group. The authors point out that repair avoided the costs and morbidity associated with later colostomy closure.

At the time this study was done, prospective, randomized clinical trials were few and far between. Colon injuries were usually managed based on individual preference or edicts from senior surgeons or department chairs. Obligatory colostomy was standard treatment for all but the most minimal colon injuries. There were few uniform standards for trauma care across the United States, and published reports usually consisted of selective patients from single institutions.

Much has changed in the management of colon injury since this article was published nearly four decades ago. Our resuscitation regimens have improved. Antimicrobials are more effective and criteria for their optimal use have been defined. The American Association for the Surgery of Trauma (AAST) has published a colon injury severity scale, which has provided a platform to compare results across institutions. We now treat most colon injuries with primary repair or resection with anastomosis, and the most severely injured undergo damage control laparotomy with definitive treatment delayed until the patient's condition has improved.

What makes this article so important? First, it was a prospective, randomized trial that was novel for most studies done in the 1970s. Second, the criteria for eligibility were defined and designed to exclude patients who were thought to be at risk for complications and death. Third, the outcomes measured were clearly important both for patients and surgeons. Fourth, the results were presented at a prestigious surgical meeting and published in a highly respected peer-reviewed journal.

Elegant is often used to describe clinical trials. This one was elegant for its time and helped change attitudes and practice for colon injury management.

Editor Notes: In the early 1970s, these authors performed an important randomized clinical trial comparing ostomy with primary repair for penetrating colon injuries. This work challenged the dogma that mandated fecal diversion for any colonic injury, which was promulgated in World War II. This trial proved the safety and feasibility of immediate repair of the colon without proximal diversion in a selected group of patients (about half of wounded met the inclusion criteria). Infection risk, complications, hospitalization, and ultimately costs were reduced in the primary closure group. Subsequently, additional work expanded upon this seminal work and demonstrated that nearly all civilian colon wounds can be repaired primarily, if technically possible and the patient is physiologically stable enough to undergo the procedure.

Limitations:

Non-blinded population;
By definition a selected group of patients;
Colonic resection excluded.

CHAPTER 30

Nonoperative Salvage of Computed Tomography-Diagnosed Splenic Injuries: Utilization of Angiography for Triage and Embolization for Hemostasis

Sclafani SJ, Shaftan GW, Scalea TM, Patterson LA, Kohl L, Kantor A, Herskowitz MM, et al. J Trauma 39(5):818–825; discussion 826–827, 1995

Abstract

Objectives   The aims of this study were to determine if angiographic findings can be used to predict successful nonoperative therapy of splenic injury, and to determine if coil embolization of the proximal splenic artery provides effective hemostasis.

Methods   Splenic injuries detected by diagnostic imaging between 1981 and 1993 at a level I trauma center were prospectively collected and retrospectively reviewed after management by protocol that used diagnostic peritoneal lavage, computed tomography (CT), angiography, transcatheter embolization, and laparotomy. Computed tomography was performed initially or after positive diagnostic peritoneal lavage. Angiography was performed urgently in stabilized patients with CT-diagnosed splenic injuries. Patients without angiographic extravasation were treated by bed-rest alone; those with angiographic extravasation underwent coil embolization of the proximal splenic artery followed by bed-rest.

Results   Patients (172) with blunt splenic injury are the subject of this study. Twenty-two patients were initially managed operatively, because of associated injuries or disease (11 patients) or the surgeon was unwilling to attempt nonoperative therapy (11 patients) and decided to perform a splenectomy (17 patients) or splenorrhaphy (5 patients). One hundred fifty of 172 consecutive patients (87%) with CT-diagnosed splenic injury were stable enough to be considered for nonoperative management. Eighty-seven of the 90 patients managed by bed-rest alone, and 56 of 60 patients treated by splenic artery occlusion and bed-rest had a successful outcome. Overall, splenic salvage was 88%. It was 97% among those managed nonoperatively, including 61 grade III and grade IV splenic injuries. Sixty percent of patients received no blood transfusions. Three of 150 patients treated nonoperatively underwent delayed splenectomy for infarction (one patient) or splenic infection (two patients).

Conclusions   (1) Hemodynamically stable patients with splenic injuries of all grades and no other indications for laparotomy can often be managed nonoperatively, especially when the injury is further characterized by arteriography. (2) The absence of contrast extravasation on splenic arteriography seems to be a reliable predictor of successful nonoperative management. We suggest its use to triage CT-diagnosed splenic injuries to bed-rest or intervention. (3) Coil embolization of the proximal splenic artery is an effective method of hemostasis in stabilized patients with splenic injury. It expands the number of patients who can be managed nonoperatively.

Author Commentary by Salvatore J.A. Sclafani

In 1966, *The Fantastic Voyage*, a cinematic portrait of lifesaving treatment by a "miniaturized" medical team in a submarine injected into an antecubital vein, was the teenage inspiration for a young radiologist to explore endovascular techniques of traumatic hemorrhage control. In 1978 at Brooklyn's Kings County Hospital, a patient with intrasplenic hemorrhage was referred for diagnostic arteriography. The radiologist wanted to help the surgeon by preoperatively controlling bleeding using gelfoam embolization. Instead, he was upbraided by the senior surgeon for wasting an opportunity to explore splenorrhaphy, a new treatment for splenic salvage.

The patient was observed but infection resulted in splenectomy. When the radiologist apologized, Gerald Shaftan, Chief of Trauma Surgery and my mentor, smiled and said, "Go figure out a better way." The subsequent collaboration resulted in the first publication in 1981 of three methods of endovascular treatment for splenic injury[1] and culminated with the first large series presented in 1995 at a major trauma meeting.[2] Based on splenic artery ligation used to salvage spleens of two children[3] and on advancements in computed tomography for nonoperative diagnosis,[4] splenic artery embolization (SAE) became our preferred method of hemorrhage control for stabilized patients with splenic injury and hemoperitoneum.

Resistance was strong within our group, but stronger within the national and international trauma communities. Some radiologists and surgeons asserted that there was no role for angiography in acute trauma. "Patients would die in X-ray." "Only Sclafani would come in at night." At a national meeting, "The lunatic fringe in Brooklyn is at it again." How a few decades changes attitudes! SAE has been accepted as a standard of care.

Resistance to innovation is common: antibiotics for ulcers, angioplasty for peripheral vascular disease, the Earth revolving around the sun, to name a few. My search to understand why innovation can take so long led me to Gustav Fleck[5] and Thomas Kuhn,[6] both physicians/philosophers, who provided a rationale:

Science requires seminal ideas by luminaries. Those who embrace these ideas form groups to elaborate concepts, set initiatives, create values, develop methodologies, and invent instruments to validate the "truth" of the seminal ideas. According to Kuhn, *conventional* science validates and esteems its originators, building upon their work to create a society of like-minded individuals and groups who have a standard, a culture, and bond related to that seminal work. Student learns from teacher. Conventional wisdom becomes like a religion. The society is very loyal to its roots.

Science becomes *radical* when evolving technology uncovers new truths, when old observations cannot be explained by the evidence, or when former algorithms do not provide solutions. Often radical change occurs simply because the society at-large demands it. Those paradigm shifts often require outsiders who think differently, yet who are able to break through the conventional and alter the conceptions of the group.

My mentor was an iconoclast who enjoyed looking *outside* the box. Without his encouragement and without my reaching *into* trauma circles, the fantasies of a young man might not have been realized.

REFERENCES

1. Sclafani SJA. The role of angiographic hemostasis in salvage of the injured spleen. *Radiology.* 1981; 141: 645–650.
2. Sclafani SJA, Shaftan GW, Scalea TM, Patterson LA, Kohl L, Kantor A, et al. Nonoperative salvage of computed tomography diagnosed splenic injuries: Utilization of angiography for triage and embolization for hemostasis. *J Trauma.* 1995; 39: 818–827.
3. Keramidas DC. The ligation of the spenic artery in the treatment of traumatic rupture of the spleen. *Surgery.* 1979; 85: 530–533.
4. Federle MP, Goldberg HI, Kaiser JA, Moss AA, Jeffrey, Jr RB, Mall JC. Evaluation of abdominal trauma by computed tomography. *Radiology.* 1981; 138: 637–644.
5. Fleck L. *Genesis and Development of a Scientific Fact.* Chicago, IL: University of Chicago Press; 1979. (Translation of original 1935 Schwabe & Co. Basel, Switzerland)
6. Kuhn TS. *The Structure of Scientific Revolutions.* Chicago, IL: University of Chicago Press; 1962.

Expert Commentary by Ali Salim

It is obvious to all practicing trauma surgeons that nonoperative management of blunt splenic injury in hemodynamically stable patients is the standard of care. This was not always the case. Operative intervention for all injuries was routine. But with the advancement of computed tomography (CT), a reliable method for identifying intra-abdominal injuries and causes of hemoperitoneum, nonoperative management of splenic injuries became more routine. However, it was not until the introduction of angiography and angiographic embolization that nonoperative management became the standard of care. Now with angiographic embolization, intervening when active bleeding was identified was now possible.

This historic paper by Sclafani et al. set the stage of what was truly possible, by not only identifying splenic injuries, which were actively bleeding, but intervening and thereby improving the likelihood of avoiding a splenectomy. As nonoperative management became the standard of care, so too did the use of angioembolization as an adjunct to nonoperative management.

It is fascinating to look back and see how much of this paper foreshadowed what is current practice today. This study accomplished two things: first to assess for contrast extravasation from the injured spleen, and second to evaluate if splenic artery coil embolization would be effective in these patients with extravasation. CT scan use in trauma was still in its infancy and contrast extravasation was not at all apparent on the first-generation CT scans. Identifying contrast extravasation as a marker of a continued bleed and a potential indication for embolization was quite novel. Interestingly, it also raised the question that still has not been answered over 20 years later: Do we need to embolize all patients with evidence of contrast extravasation?[1,2]

The role of angiographic embolization is better defined today.[3] At our center, angiographic embolization is reserved for hemodynamically stable patients with high-grade injuries (IV and V) and evidence of contrast extravasation on CT. The success of angiographic embolization has also been useful in nontraditional settings: hemodynamically labile patients with solid organ injuries[4] and even in the nonoperative management of penetrating solid organ injuries.[5]

Nonoperative management of splenic injuries was already becoming a common practice for hemodynamically stable patients. This paper helped push the envelope by widening the number of patients eligible for nonoperative management, but also improving its success rate. Today, angioembolization is an important adjunct for the management of trauma patients and has become a requirement to maintain high level trauma verification status. Not a small feat from a group of dedicated trauma surgeons and radiologists practicing at a county hospital in Brooklyn.

REFERENCES

1. Olthof DC, van der Vlies CH, Joose P, et al. Consensus strategies for the nonoperative management of patients with blunt splenic injury: A Delphi study. *J Trauma Acute Care Surg.* 2013; 74: 1567–1574.
2. Watson GA, Hoffman MK, Peitzman AB. Nonoperative management of blunt splenic injury: What is new? *Eur J Trauma Emerg Surg.* 2015; 41: 219–228.
3. Stassen NA, Bhullar I, Cheng JD, et al. Selective nonoperative management of blunt splenic injury: An Eastern association for the surgery of trauma practice management guideline. *J Trauma Acute Care Surg.* 2012; 73: S294–S300.
4. Hagiwara A, Fukushima H, Murata A, et al. Blunt splenic injury: Usefulness of transcatheter arterial embolization in patients with a transient response to fluid resuscitation. *Radiology.* 205; 235: 57–64.
5. Demetriades D, Hadjizacharia P, Constantinou C, et al. Selective nonoperative management of penetrating abdominal solid organ injuries. *Ann Surg.* 2006; 244: 620–628.

Editor Notes: This was one of the first reports to describe the value of angiographic embolization in arresting hemorrhage from splenic injury. Sixty of 172 patients with splenic trauma were embolized, and 56/60 had a successful outcome.

Limitations:

Retrospective review;

No rigid management protocols (22 patients were explored at the discretion of the surgeon);

Patients undergoing angio were highly selected;

No control group so unclear as to impact of angioembolization.

CHAPTER 31

Arteriography in the Management of Hemorrhage from Pelvic Fractures

Margolies MN, Ring EJ, Waltman AC, Kerr WS Jr, Baum S.
N Engl J Med 287(7):317–321, 1972

Abstract   Localization of the source of massive hemorrhage from pelvic fractures is not often made clinically, and the results of expectant management or of hypogastric artery ligation are frequently unsatisfactory. Three patients with pelvic fractures and rapid blood loss were examined by transfemoral aortography. In all of them, bleeding originated from obturator artery branches in the vicinity of fractures involving the pubic rami. In two of these patients, hemorrhage was controlled by selective catheterization of the anterior division of the hypogastric artery, followed by injection of autologous clotted blood.

Arterial bleeding from pelvic fractures may be more common than has previously been supposed. Arteriographic localization of the bleeding site should improve selection of patients for surgical exploration when the described method of hemostasis fails.

Author Commentary by Michael N. Margolies

Hemorrhage is the major contributing factor in mortality among patients with pelvic fractures. Prior to this report (1972), the prevailing dictum stated that bleeding from major pelvic fractures was venous in origin. Evidence from "static" postmortem studies was unrevealing, except in the case of tears of the major iliac veins. Inasmuch as surgical exploration aimed at controlling bleeding directly, or bilateral internal iliac artery ligation, seldom succeeded, an "expectant" approach had been recommended in the somewhat vain hope that hemorrhage would abate, owing to tamponade.

At that time, there were few hospitals in the United States with dedicated trauma units. Computed tomographic imaging was not used in clinical practice. Arteriography (and venography) were the only available "dynamic" diagnostic methods capable of localizing bleeding.

The use of arteriography to control hemorrhage occurred through serendipity. I was a neophyte general surgeon "on-call" for the emergency ward at Massachusetts General Hospital. That institution had just recruited Stanley Baum from the University of Pennsylvania, a pioneer in arteriographic diagnosis and control of gastrointestinal bleeding and who arrived with the necessary radiologic equipment. Faced with three patients with massive bleeding from pelvic fractures over the course of 12 days in 1971, we raised the question whether there was an identifiable arterial bleeding site by selective arteriography. Each of these patients was bleeding from the obturator artery in the vicinity of fractures of the pubic rami. Intra-arterial infusion of posterior pituitary extract, useful in controlling gastrointestinal bleeding, proved ineffective. Dr. Baum proposed using selective intra-arterial autologous clotted blood as a therapeutic "embolism." In two of the three cases in which this could be achieved technically, post-injection arteriography demonstrated that extravasation of dye had ceased and clinical bleeding abated promptly. Subsequent series of patients confirmed the efficacy of this approach. In the intervening years, advances in interventional radiology often eclipsed advances in surgery.

Arteriographic control was achieved relatively late in the course of these patients who often sustained multiple injuries. We proposed that arteriography be undertaken early in those patients with significant ongoing bleeding, in the absence of an intra-abdominal bleeding site, in order to avoid the pernicious effects of massive transfusion. It is gratifying that arterial localization of pelvic bleeding site(s) with attendant embolization, has continued to be of therapeutic use in the care of patients with these most challenging of traumatic injuries.

Expert Commentary by Kevin S. Hirsch

In the practice of medicine, a significant portion of what is currently known is fallacy. However, new concepts of treatment emerge, and some pioneers enable those concepts to blossom into incontrovertible truths. These truths can result in a complete paradigm shift leading to entirely new areas of specialization that impact the lives of patients worldwide. This is the case of the landmark 1972 article "Arteriography in the management of hemorrhage from pelvic fractures" by Drs. Margolies, Ring, Waltman, Kerr, and Baum. What is now routine in the care of trauma patients was spurred by this small group of physicians who translated the theoretical into the practical. At the time, the concept of transcatheter embolization for control of hemorrhage was very limited with embolization for GI bleeding first described by Rosch and Dotter[1] in February 1972. Dr. Baum extrapolated the concept of embolization for GI bleeding by utilizing autologous clotted venous blood and applied it to traumatic pelvic vascular injuries. The result was an elegant, minimally invasive approach to access and treat the sources of life-threatening, poorly controlled pelvic hemorrhage.

The report of treatment of three patients with transcatheter embolization was a vast step forward for Interventional Radiology (IR) and has led to a potent partnership between Trauma Surgery and IR for the care of trauma patients. The principles of embolization are foundational and underlie broad areas of IR in the care of traumatic injury[2] as well as a multitude of other diseases such as uterine fibroids, hepatic and other metastases, vascular malformations, neuro-intervention, and many others. An entire industry has been built around embolization and embolic agents have evolved. Early attempts were made to modify autologous clots[3] without considerable success. Surgical gelatin (Gelfoam; Upjohn, Kalamazoo, MI) became the embolization material of choice[4] and continues to be the only widely used temporary embolic. Permanent embolics have evolved from very early use of liquid embolics such as isobutyl 2-cyanoacrylate to modern N-butyl-2 cyanoacrylate and others. Permanent embolic particles have advanced from polyvinyl alcohol particles in 1974 to trisacryl gelatin and other modern microspheres. Embolic coils were introduced in 1975[5] and continue to play an important role in embolization. In addition, occlusion balloons have expanded from the IR suite to the trauma bay with the use of Resuscitative Endovascular Balloon Occlusion of the Aorta (REBOA).

Traumatic vascular injuries of all types in nearly all locations of the body can now be treated with the same basic principles of transcatheter embolization. As techniques have progressed, so has the multidisciplinary approach. Modern trauma centers have capabilities both in the IR suite as well as hybrid angiography/operating rooms. Stable patients can be easily treated in the IR suite while hybrid operating rooms enable less stable patients to be cared for by multidisciplinary teams. IR now routinely collaborates with trauma surgery, orthopedic surgery, hepatobiliary surgery, urology, obstetrics and gynecology, and others. The result is a marked reduction in hemorrhage and improved care for patients with traumatic injury and beyond. We owe a great debt to these visionary physicians that should be repaid by continuing the work to advance the field.

REFERENCES

1. Rosch J, Dotter CT, Brown MJ. Selective arterial embolization: A new method for control of acute gastrointestinal bleeding. *Radiology*. 1972; 102: 303–306.
2. Zealley IA, Chakraverty S. The role of interventional radiology in trauma. *BMJ*. 2010; 340: 356–360. doi:10.1136/bmj.c497.
3. Bookstein JJ, Closta EM, Foley D, Walter JF. Transcatheter hemostasis of gastrointestinal bleeding using modified autogenous clot. *Radiology*. 1974; 113: 277–285.
4. Golf RE, Grace DM. Gelfoam embolization of the left gastric artery for bleeding ulcer: Experimental considerations. *Radiology*. 1975; 116: 575–580.
5. Gianturco C, Anderson JH, Wallace S. Mechanical devices for arterial occlusion. *Am J Roentgenol Radium Ther Nucl Med*. 1975; 124(3): 428–435.

Editor Notes: These authors provide one of the first descriptions of the successful early use of angiographic embolization for termination of bleeding after pelvic fractures.

Limitations:

Only three cases presented;
Technique only addressed arterial bleeding.

CHAPTER 32

Early versus Delayed Stabilization of Femoral Fractures: A Prospective Randomized Study

Bone LB, Johnson KD, Weigelt J, Scheinberg R. J Bone Joint Surg Am 71(3):336–340, 1989

Abstract A prospective randomized study comparing the results of early with delayed reduction and stabilization of acute femoral fractures in adults was performed over a 2-year period in 178 patients. Only patients who were more than 65 years old and had a fracture of the hip were excluded. Arterial blood gases, injury-severity score at the time of admission, pulmonary function, days in the hospital, days in the intensive care unit, and hospital costs were recorded for all patients. The patients were divided into two groups: those who had an isolated fracture of the femur and those who had multiple injuries. When stabilization of the fracture was delayed in the patients who had multiple injuries, the incidence of pulmonary complications (adult respiratory-distress syndrome, fat embolism, and pneumonia) was higher, the hospital stay was longer, and the number of days in the intensive care unit was increased. The cost of hospital care showed a statistically significant increase for all patients who had delayed treatment of the fracture, compared with those who had early stabilization.

Author Commentary by John A. Weigelt

Early fracture fixation has become a standard of care that few doubt today. At the time this article was published, the data were less than robust. The majority were retrospective reviews that were still questioned by many. Dr. Larry Bone, a young orthopedist, was influenced by Dr. John Border who felt that protracted bed-rest was bad. We agreed and felt that early fixation of femoral fractures would decrease the morbidity associated with this major long bone fracture. This common theme produced a collegial effort to conduct this prospective study.

While the definitions of respiratory failure have morphed since this study was published, the results have not. Fixation of femoral fractures within the first 24 hours is no longer debated. It is easy to look at early fixation as the major advance, but I suggest that these results helped us change our thought process about the effect immobilization has on our patients.

I clearly remember at the time of this study having injured patients in traction awaiting their orthopedic procedure on our trauma wards. Their care was difficult for nurses and physicians. Pulmonary complications were common, and many of these patients ended up in the intensive care unit, not for their initial injuries but for their pneumonia, respiratory failure, or decubitus ulcers secondary to their prolonged bed-rest. While it did not happen overnight, traction did disappear in favor of early operative stabilization. Truly a benefit for patients and caregivers.

It is gratifying to see the principles set forth in this 1989 paper continue to be applied in the management of our critically ill patients with or without orthopedic injuries. Early mobilization is practiced throughout the hospital, even extending to medical patients. This helps decrease pulmonary complications, venous-thrombotic events, and deconditioning, and speeds recovery. While it has taken some time, early fracture stabilization now extends to spinal column fractures with very similar results. Tracing these changes to one paper is always suspect, but certainly this paper should be identified as helping start a very positive movement in our management approaches to the injured patient.

Drs. Bone and Johnson were the orthopedic workhorses who pushed to get patients to the operating room early. Not an easy task when the usual care was to slip these patients in whenever time permitted. The effective team was completed by the trauma/critical care surgeons who provided the daily patient care. As I reflect on this intervention for patients with femur fractures, it really produced a beneficial effect for a much greater patient population. Our premise was correct, but I believe none of us had considered the "halo" effect we observed.

REFERENCES

Bliemel C, Lefering R, Buecking B, et al. Early or delayed stabilization in severely injured patients with spinal fractures? Current surgical objectivity according to the Trauma Registry of DGU: Treatment of spine injuries in polytrauma patients. *J Trauma Acute Care Surg*. 2014; 76(2): 366–373.

Epstein NE. A review article on the benefits of early mobilization following spinal surgery and other medical/surgical procedures. *Surg Neurol Int*. 2014; 5: S66.

Park K, Park Y, Sep W, et al. Clinical results of early stabilization of spine fractures in polytrauma patients. *J Crit Care*. 2014; 29(4): 694e7–694e9.

Expert Commentary by Hans-Christoph Pape

Bone's study caused a sustained change in the management of long bone fractures. Prior to his work, the patient with a major fracture was thought to be too sick to be surgically stabilized. The major fear among surgeons in the 1960s and 1970s was the development of the *fat embolism syndrome*, which has a clinical presentation resembling adult respiratory distress syndrome (ARDS).

It was thought to be caused by fat emboli from the bone after fracture. The idea of having the patient wait in traction was that, over a period of 7–10 days, the showers of fat emboli had been cleared. The clinical picture of fat embolism syndrome consisted of pulmonary dysfunction and cerebral dysfunction. It was diagnosed by detecting fat emboli in the retina and/or in the bloodstream (Gurd test). When artificial ventilation became a standard treatment, the pulmonary dysfunction could be overcome or delayed.

Therefore, the standard treatment for major fractures was to perform traction for temporary fixation for about a week after admission. In the late 1970s and early 1980s, several trauma centers began to perform earlier definitive fixation, in part due to availability of ventilator support. Before Bone's study, there were three retrospective studies that reported less pulmonary failure when early stabilization of major fractures, namely the femur shaft, was performed. Two of these (Riska et al. and Goris et al.) were from different centers in Europe and the third was by Ken Johnson, who later became coauthor in LB Bone's series performed at Parkland Memorial Hospital.

The prospective, randomized trial then performed by Bone and Johnson had some spectacular logistical details. Not only did they randomize patients with femur fractures, but they also documented cardiovascular details along with the development of organ dysfunction and were able to provide detailed information because of daily standardized blood gas values. They used standardized criteria for blood gas withdrawal and took care of all open fractures in the operating room. Also, they separated those patients that sustained isolated femur fractures from those that had multiple injuries.

They were able to include 95 patients with isolated fractures and 83 multiply injured patients and found that the ones with multiple injuries had lower rates of ARDS, pulmonary function, and fat emboli. The concept became accepted worldwide.

Decades later, some centers began to stabilize all fractures rather than just the major ones, thinking that the duration and magnitude of surgery does not play a role. Therefore, a slight modification to the role of early total care of major fractures was performed by using external fixateurs in very sick patients (damage control concept).

In summary, Bone and Johnson's study set the pace toward the most important change in the management of trauma patients with extremity fractures since the beginning of surgical treatment of bone injuries. It has remained an important and standardized treatment in all patients with major fractures ever since this groundbreaking proof of a new strategy of surgical management.

Editor Notes: This important study suggested that early operative stabilization of femur fractures in multiply injured patients minimized pulmonary complications and shortened the length of ICU and hospital stay.

Limitations:

Heterogeneous population with moderate number (n = 83) of multiply injured;
Study excluded patients over 65 years of age;
The clinicians were not blinded as to the patient group when making decisions on ICU stay;
Arterial blood gases were obtained just once per day and the primary difference in pulmonary complications was the number of abnormally low arterial blood gases.

CHAPTER 33

The Use of Temporary Vascular Shunts as a Damage Control Adjunct in the Management of Wartime Vascular Injury

Rasmussen TE, Clouse WD, Jenkins DH, Peck MA, Eliason JL, Smith DL. J Trauma 61(1):8–12; discussion 12–15, 2006

Abstract

Background While the use of vascular shunts as a damage control adjunct has been described in series from civilian institutions no contemporary military experience has been reported. The objective of this study is to examine patterns of use and effectiveness of temporary vascular shunts in the contemporary management of wartime vascular injury.

Materials From September 1, 2004 to August 31, 2005, 2,473 combat injuries were treated at the Central Echelon III surgical facility in Iraq. Vascular injuries were entered into a registry and reviewed. Location of shunts was divided into proximal and distal, and shunt patency, complications and limb viability were examined.

Results There were 126 extremity vascular injuries treated. Fifty-three (42%) had been operated on at forward locations, and 30 of 53 (57%) had temporary shunts in place upon arrival to our facility. The patency for shunts in proximal vascular injuries was 86% (n = 22), compared with 12% (n = 8) for distal shunts (p < 0.05). All shunts placed in proximal venous injuries were patent (n = 4). Systemic heparin was not used, and there were no shunt complications. All shunted injuries were reconstructed with vein in theatre, and early viability for extremities in which shunts were used was 92%.

Conclusions Temporary vascular shunts are common in the management of wartime vascular injury. Shunts in proximal injuries including veins have high patency rates, compared with those placed in distal injuries. This vascular adjunct represents a safe and effective damage control technique and is preferable to attempted reconstruction in austere conditions.

Author Commentary by W. Darrin Clouse

This manuscript was conceived surrounding our initial experiences with the theater care structure in Operation Iraqi Freedom. The Joint Theater Trauma

System/Registry (JTTS/JTTR) was maturing, and the proof of Forward Surgical Team (FST; level II care) strategic viability was burgeoning. Our approach to vascular injury management needed definition. Specifically, compared to World War II and the Vietnam War, the last two major conflicts involving the United States, early, forward arterial and venous injury delineation was now possible but definitive reconstruction impractical.

We found ourselves quickly absorbing conceptual history as well as prior reported experiences with temporary vascular shunts (TVS) for injury. Since Vietnam, 30 years more experience with vascular surgery had occurred, and daily shunt use with carotid surgery was commonplace. Military preparations for mass casualty or the next conflict regularly included discussion of shunt use for temporization. Now, it was time to put these notions into action, and level II centers were using TVS and moving casualties on expeditiously to comprehensive level III theater care at Combat Surgical Hospitals (CSHs) and the Air Force Theater Hospital (AFTH). Assessment of the approach was needed.

Several foundational impressions came from this small case series from theater. First, use of TVS could indeed be successful in early limb perfusion during war. This was the groundwork for later analysis describing not only limb salvage benefits, but also animal work that defined benefits of TVS with regard to ischemic time and physiologic perturbations. Essentially, this illuminated the way forward and provided a clinical needs assessment toward better understanding of TVS for use in military and civilian extremity vascular injury.

Next, TVS was best utilized with injuries proximally in extremities. It became clear that TVS use beyond the elbow or trifurcation was not necessary. Frankly, it's difficult in these locations and doesn't affect limb salvage except possibly in rare, select circumstances. The notion that systemic anticoagulation was not needed with shunts in place was supported. This was not earth shattering, as animal studies had indicated such. Yet, this confirmed that in humans, TVS largely do remain open without it. This simple feature reassured those caring for the injured with a litany of reasons to avoid anticoagulation. Finally, communication that evacuation and patient movement with shunts in place could be effectively accomplished was an important message.

The manuscript provided kindling in delineating posture for vascular injury care in Operation Iraqi Freedom (OIF) and ultimately also in Operation Enduring Freedom (OEF). New US military guidelines on extremity vascular injury within the context of modern theater trauma systems and forward care were created. Seemingly the culmination of efforts focused on easy, early reperfusion, starting in the 1900s and World War I, through experiences in Europe, Israel, and small civilian reports, this report of 30 plastic tubes placed into vessel injuries then evacuated in a war established a mindset. The dictum of "vascular damage control" built on early, temporary perfusion restoration (TVS), fasciotomy, embolectomy, and only regional heparin became common vernacular.

REFERENCES

Gifford SM, Aidinian G, Clouse WD, et al. Effect of temporary shunting on extremity vascular injury: An outcome analysis from the global war on terror vascular injury initiative. *J Vasc Surg.* 2009; 50(3): 549–556.

Hancock H, Rasmussen TE, Walker AJ, et al. History of temporary intravascular shunts in the management of vascular injury. *J Vasc Surg.* 2010; 52: 1405–1409.

Hancock H, Stannard A, Burkhardt GE, et al. Hemorrhagic shock worsens neuromuscular recovery in a porcine model of hind limb vascular injury and ischemia-reperfusion. *J Vasc Surg.* 2011; 53: 1052–1062.

Expert Commentary by Jeffrey H. Lawson

The paper by Rasmussen et al. characterizes use of vascular shunts in the setting of military trauma to assist with expedited vascular control and perfusion of acutely damaged vessels in austere conditions. This paper highlights a relatively large clinical experience of vascular shunts that were used to stabilize perfusion of both upper and lower extremities in acute and mass casualty settings. The authors report on the use of vascular shunts in 30 of 126 extremity vascular injuries over a 12-month period between 2004 and 2005 during the Operation Iraqi Freedom campaign with early extremity viability rate (limb salvage) of 92%. The paper provides a reasonable experience and thoughtful discussion of the use of vascular shunts to assist with emergent limb salvage in the setting of military trauma.

Vascular shunts have been used in cardiovascular surgery and trauma for over 50 years. The most common application, with the largest clinical experience, is its use during carotid endarterectomy. While the use of shunts to preserve brain perfusion during carotid endarterectomy is still debated among various segments of the vascular community, there is no question among those who are adept at using shunts that they find this a reassuring asset to address complex carotid interventions. Over the past 50 years, the use of vascular shunts has evolved to include trauma and other modes of vascular reconstruction. As noted in this paper, the first use of vascular shunts in combat-related injuries was published by Eger et al. in 1971 during the Vietnam War and, prior to the Rasmussen et al. publication, was the only significant experience reporting vascular shunt use in a combat environment.

One interesting use of vascular shunts described in this paper is the potential to address acute venous injury. It is this author's opinion, the current practice among vascular/trauma surgeons, is to ligate the venous injury instead of attempting repair. In this study, all of the venous shunts attempted (4), remained patent, and allowed for venous drainage of the injured extremity until definitive repair could be accomplished. Further, while conventional wisdom argues that most venous shunts will thrombose, none of the ones reported in this series appeared to undergo that complication, which begs the question, should we be shunting and reconstructing more venous injuries?

This study also explores the use of shunts in the distal extremity circulation (below the knee or elbow). While it appears that no adverse limb salvage events occurred in the distal shunts attempted, the authors observed a very high rate of shunt thrombosis. While shunt attempts in this subgroup are noble, this observation suggests that the vessel could have just as easily been ligated with potentially the same outcome. Until small caliber, non-thrombotic shunts become available, it appears that shunting distal vessels may be technically possible, but an unwarranted use of critical time and resource in the setting of combat injury.

Finally, it is noted in the paper that none of the patients in this study were treated with systemic anticoagulation therapy following shunt placement and transport. It is also remarkable that the reported transport times to definitive care were often as short as only a few hours. It is also unclear what role trauma induced coagulopathies may play in the need for early or therapeutic anticoagulation use during transport. With only anecdotal experience, there is clearly no consensus on the use of anticoagulation following shunt placement; however, this author might recommend some low-dose heparin therapy if the shunt is projected to be in place more than 8 hours and continuous pulse oximetry monitoring of the distal extremity during the transport process.

From this paper, I would conclude that the use of vascular shunts during the damage control or transport phases of care is a useful option to assist with limb salvage in austere environments and should remain a surgical option in forward operating units.

Editor Notes: This was an important study demonstrating the value of intravascular shunts in wartime. One hundred twenty-six extremity vascular injuries underwent placement of shunts. No complications were noted, and the patency rates were extremely high. This paper led to the widespread use of shunts in the care of both combat and civilian trauma victims with vascular injuries.

Limitations:

Small series;
No control group;
Limited follow-up data;
Relationship to amputation unclear (7% had amputation);
And most shunts were <2-hour duration.

CHAPTER 34

Endovascular Stent Grafts and Aortic Rupture: A Case Series

Karmy-Jones R, Hoffer E, Meissner MH, Nicholls S,
Mattos M. J Trauma 55(5):805–810, 2003

Abstract   The paper by Karmy-Jones was among the earliest, if not the first, to report a series of 11 trauma patients with thoracic aortic injuries treated with percutaneously inserted endografts.[1] Despite the small size of this series, this paper addressed most of the subsequent concerns relating to aortic endografts: migration of stent, endoleaks, infection, obliteration of the orifice of the left subclavian artery, and access site issues of iliac artery injury, as well as size, length, and configuration of the endograft. Significant debate relative to long-term complications of migration and dilatation continued for several years after the publication of Dr. Karmy-Jones's classic article. Those complications are not now being reported.

Background   Endovascular stent grafts (EVSGs) offer an alternative in the management of traumatic rupture of the aorta, particularly in patients who are at prohibitive operative risk.

Methods   We conducted a retrospective review of 11 cases managed by EVSGs over a 4-year period. EVSGs were defined as "noncommercial" (graft material hand sewn over metallic stents) or "commercial" (grafts marketed for infrarenal aortic or thoracic aneurysms). Data collected included the difference between endovascular stent graft length, tear length (apposition length), and location relative to the left subclavian artery.

Results   EVSGs (three noncommercial and eight commercial, including AneuRx cuff [six], Talent [one], and Ancure aortic tube graft [one]) were used in 11 patients. Six were placed less than or equal to 8 hours from injury, one after 14 hours, three after 5 days, and one 10 years after injury. Routes of access included femoral (four), iliac (three), and abdominal aorta (four). Average landing zone diameter was 18.8 ± 3.5 mm, distance from the left subclavian artery was 2.85 ± 2.1 cm, and tear length was 1.54 ± 1.0 cm. In four cases, the apposition length was less than 2 cm. There were two cases of persistent endoleak, and two cases of endoleak noted and treated at deployment. Persistent endoleak occurred in two of three noncommercial EVSGs. Endoleak occurred in three of four cases when apposition length was less than 2 cm, one of which was treated successfully at the time of placement by deploying extension grafts. Endoleak occurred in two of six cases when deployment was within 2 cm of the origin of the left subclavian artery. In one case of persistent endoleak, open repair was performed 3 weeks later when the patient had stabilized. Ultimately, there were three deaths, two caused by severe closed head injury and one caused by respiratory failure.

Conclusions   Endovascular stent grafts can be placed emergently. Commercial grafts result in better results than noncommercial grafts. Available "cuff extenders" are sufficient for the majority of aortic injuries but often require deployment via the iliac or aorta because of the shorter delivery system. Tears more than 1.5 cm resulting in apposition length less than 2 cm or those near or in the curvature of the aorta are associated with increased endoleak risk. The ideal thoracic EVSG would be available in 5-, 7.5-, 10-, and 15-cm lengths and mounted on a system 80 cm in length.

Author Commentary by Riyad Karmy-Jones

The paper was written at a time when thoracic specific devices were not widely available, and those that were, were designed for aneurysmal disease. It was also a time of struggle both within and without the vascular community as to who would "control" these emerging technologies.

This series constituted patients who were critically ill and could not be repaired by open techniques. This high-risk group was in contradistinction to many European and Canadian studies, which limited thoracic endovascular aortic repair (TEVAR) to stable patients with small injuries.

The paper reviewed the specific anatomic concerns relative to TEVAR and compared "off-the-shelf" constructed stents to commercially available abdominal grafts. With reference to the left subclavian and stroke risk, we suggested that in young patients, the subclavian could be covered. Now we know this is true, although older patients may be at increased risk, as much from wire manipulation in the arch as impacting vertebral perfusion. Newer approaches, including fenestration and kissing stents, permit preservation of the left subclavian with greater ease. We mentioned sizing "10%–20%" (although in Table 2 we erroneously stated ">20% oversizing"). We now know that oversizing can lead to increased endocollapse. We also know that in patients with a pliable aorta, if in shock, aortic diameters can increase by as much as 30%, which requires some judgement as to appropriate sizing. We stressed the need to try and avoid lack of apposition along the inner wall and discussed "ballooning the endograft." Nowadays, we rarely do this as we are concerned about creating a dissection. Later studies confirm that the point of curvature has the maximal stress in the aorta, and if any endograft "juts up away from the inner wall," there is increased likelihood of collapse. We noted that all of us were awaiting more thoracic specific devices, including those with smaller diameters and perhaps shorter lengths. Now, we have longer delivery systems, smaller sheath sizes permitting percutaneous access, and more flexible endografts to fit the aortic curvature (with much lower incidence of lack of wall apposition). We are still waiting for shorter endografts to become more available. However, the current devices are so much more stable and predictable in deployment that the use of adenosine is rarely required. The paper also presaged the hybrid room and the occasional uses of TEVAR as a bridge to definite management (especially in younger patients).

Much has been clarified. Medical management is accepted in specific patients and is associated with an improved outcome if intervention is required. TEVAR has become the favored approach, offering a less morbid option than open repair, which tends to be relegated to ascending and arch of the aorta (although that will soon change). It appears that TEVAR is as durable as open repair, and the majority of any complications are managed percutaneously. Procedures are performed in hybrid suites, with percutaneous approaches, and can be combined with other procedures. In patients deemed to have increased risk of stroke, percutaneous approaches are available to preserve vertebral perfusion.

Expert Commentary by Kenneth L. Mattox

For several decades, emergency operation for blunt injury to the descending thoracic aorta was considered one of the biggest challenges in the fields of thoracic and trauma surgery, as well as surgical critical care and interventional radiology.[2] Strategies in prevention, diagnosis, and timing and type of operation were the subjects of many reports in the respective literature.[3] Preoperative death from free rupture of the aortic injury into the mediastinum and pleural cavity led to pharmacologic lowering of the blood pressure and sheer/stress factors on the aortic wall prior to operative control.[4] These strategies predated the introduction of CT scanning. Postinjury and postoperative complications of death, paralysis, dysphagia, infection, and pseudoaneurysm formation were constant concerns.[5]

Two quantum innovative technologies, the introduction of computed tomography scanning (CT scans) and percutaneous insertion of aortic endografts, completely and dramatically changed the diagnosis, therapeutic approaches, and outcomes of this complex injury.[1,6]

Since the publication of this article, several large series have been published, particularly from Memphis and Los Angeles.[7,8] These have confirmed and supported the initial report by Karmy-Jones. In 2017 (14 years later), the companies that are manufacturing aortic endografts have produced more compatible designs and size options. The endograft and access site complications have significantly lessened. Publications relating to any indication for an open repair of a blunt thoracic aortic injury have not emerged. Despite early predictions of long-term late complications requiring reoperation, these have not been reported.

REFERENCES

1. Fabian TC. Roger T. Sherman. Lecture: Advances in the management of blunt thoracic aortic injury—Parmley to the present. *Am Surg.* 2009; 75: 273.
2. Parmley LF, Mattingly TW, Marian WE, et al. Nonpenetrating traumatic injury of the aorta. *Circulation.* 1958; 17: 1086.
3. von Oppell UO, Dunne TT, De Groot MK, et al. Traumatic rupture: Twenty-year meta-analysis of mortality and risk of paraplegia. *Ann Thoracic Surg.* 1994; 58: 585.
4. Verdant A. Traumatic rupture of the thoracic aorta. *Ann Thoracic Surg.* 1990; 49: 686.
5. Mattox KL, Wall MJ Jr. Historic review of blunt injury to the thoracic aorta. *Chest Surg Clin N Am.* 2000; 10: 167–182.
6. Miller FB, Richardson JD, Thomas HA. Role of CT in the diagnosis of major arterial injury after blunt thoracic trauma. *Surgery.* 1989; 106: 596.
7. Demetriades D, Velmahos CG, Scalea, T. Blunt traumatic thoracic aortic injuries: Early or delayed repair-results of an American Association for the Surgery of Trauma prospective study. *J Trauma.* 2009; 66: 267. AAST series.
8. Demetriades D, Velmahos GC, Scalea TM, et al. Operative repair or endovascular stent graft in blunt traumatic thoracic aortic injuries: results of an American Association for the Surgery of Trauma Multicenter Study. *J Trauma.* 2008; 64(3): 561–570.

Editor Notes: This was one of the first case series suggesting the feasibility of aortic stent grafts for use in the setting to traumatic aortic tears (11 cases). While endoleaks occurred, primarily in the hand-sewn grafts, no cases of delayed rupture were experienced, and there was no migration of the grafts reported. No case of paraplegia after this procedure was described. Ultimately, aortic stent grafts became the standard of care after traumatic aortic injury.

Limitations:

Small case series;
Various graft materials;
No control group.

CHAPTER 35

Open Wound Drainage versus Wound Excision in Treating the Modern Assault Rifle Wound

Fackler ML, Breteau JP, Courbil LJ, Taxit R, Glas J, Fievet JP. Surgery 105(5):576–584, 1989

Abstract   Military dogma of the past 20 years preaches that excision of all injured tissue around the path of a penetrating projectile is essential in wound treatment. To find out whether excising injured muscle surrounding a bullet path benefits healing over and above the benefit provided by a simple release of tension by incision, two groups of 90-kg swine were shot in the hind leg with a replica of the AK-74 assault rifle projectile. One group was treated by excision of injured tissue around the projectile path; in the other group, no tissue was excised. Both groups were given parenteral penicillin for 5 days, and simple gauze dressings were used to cover the wounds. No difference in healing time occurred; the wounds in both groups had closed, and no epithelial defect remained by 20–22 days. These results indicate that if provided with adequate open drainage and systemic penicillin, then the simple extremity wound caused by the modern-generation assault rifle heals as rapidly when the body's defense mechanisms handle the disrupted tissue as when an attempt is made to excise it surgically.

Expert Commentary by Norman Rich

This study by Fackler and colleagues is relatively small with only five animals in each of the two groups.

While their results are interesting, it is inappropriate to expand this into clinical recommendations. No clinical changes were enacted. They do identify the confusion with semantics, and we have discussed for years the English meaning of the French word "Debridement." Our preference has been "cleansing," which in the twenty-first century has changed to "washout." We agree to incision to remove tension and in delayed wound closure; however, in the battlefield, wound removal of devitalized tissue and foreign material helps prevent infection. The authors had no infections in either group with limited contamination, and this is unrealistic in the clinical situation. Interestingly, former Dean, Jay P. Sanford, a world-respected infectious disease expert always emphasized that it was the wound debridement as we define it, and not the antibiotics, that contributed to improved results. The authors state that they are against "aggressive" debribement and "block resection" of tissue in combat wounds, and these measures have not been utilized in more than 50 years.

Gunshot wounds are a relatively small number of combat wounded, with the majority of wounds from explosive devices of various types ranging from exploding artillery shells, mortar shells, and grenades, to mention a few. In the twenty-first century, blast from improvised explosive devices (IEDs) contributes to increased contamination and increased risk of infection in combat wounds. Currently, the Center for Critical Care Initiative at the Uniformed Services University is studying biomarkers to determine when wound closure is safe from infection or whether additional washout is required.

Expert Commentary by Donald H. Jenkins

I imagine it might be difficult for residents and new faculty trained in the past decade to understand why this seminal manuscript is so important to our care of the injured patient. I am quite pleased to try to put this into context, having been trained to do what was disproven in this study and to adopt a new technique based upon science, not upon experience. Distinguishing the current evidenced-based medicine era from the experiential-based medicine, in which I was trained, is important in this context.

I was just starting the final rotation of my internship in the USAF Hospital in San Antonio on Rich Roetger's trauma service when this article was published. As a medical student, I learned from World War II, Korean, and Vietnam veteran surgeons in the National Capital Region at Uniformed Services University about injury care on the battlefield, and this was reinforced during my trauma rotation. This included core excision of bullet tracts in the soft tissue and was often extended to excision of soft tissue around stab wound tracts as well. And now Fackler was saying all of that was unnecessary, although it was a part of our daily practice and all of my faculty had learned this practice during their training. Fackler was promoting merely linear extension of the wound to allow for adequate drainage and minimize debridement. Let's just say the article was not favorably reviewed in journal club.

Like most things in surgery, it took quite a few years to realize a change in practice based upon the solid data that Fackler provided in this study. But it did eventually take hold. Similarly, we were taught and practiced the technique of true delayed primary closure for many of these wounds and for appendectomies. Dress the wound in the operating room (OR), don't touch it again until returning to the OR 5 days later, and then close it. Never really did make sense to me, honestly.

In medical school, I was issued the US Revision of the NATO Emergency War Surgery Manual, which endorsed both of these techniques as did the 2nd revision in 1988.

It was with great pride that in the third revision, I was able to work with the esteemed editors to remove this old dogma and replace it with the work that Fackler outlined in this study. In Iraq and Afghanistan, we taught surgeons, new to combat injury, linear incision and minimal debridement with great success. Not only was it more practical, we believe it led to better functional outcomes. We also introduced negative pressure wound therapy and delayed closure of combat wounds, something cautioned against according to the old dogma.

Hopefully, you can now appreciate why the editors chose this landmark paper for inclusion in this textbook. It changed my practice, my teaching, and improved outcomes of injured combatants. Seems like a pretty good set of reasons to include Fackler's work herein.

Editor Notes: This paper reported the results of a large animal study replicating the injuries induced by military assault rifles in an effort to validate the standard practice of wound excision promulgated at the time. Surgical debridement was compared with serial dressing changes and no benefit of operative management was found. The review of the literature in this manuscript is expansive and informs the reader on why these results were actually predictable. This single article challenged the dogma of the day and changed the way penetrating high velocity wounds were managed in both the military and civilian setting.

Limitations:

Animal study;
Limited number of pigs;
Pigs were not their own control (meaning did not have two extremities injured on a single animal with one serving as a control limb);
Possible variability and bias of operating surgeons;
Lack of assessor blinding.

CHAPTER 36

Primary Excision and Grafting of Large Burns

Jackson D, Topley E, Cason JS, Lowbury EJL. Ann Surg 152(2):167–189, 1960

Abstract   This paper represents the first attempt at realizing immediate closure of large burns in an era when the rest of medical care could have been up to the task. Early closure of burn wounds has since been key to reducing hypermetabolism, cachexia, infection, and death.

Expert Commentary by David N. Herndon

Although Cope et al. had earlier described improved recovery after full-thickness burns with prompt excision and grafting, they noted that "threatening physiologic instability" was a limit to the broader application of early excision. In their series, full thickness wounds were generally excised within the first 10 days in patients with extensive burns, with excision of up to 12% of the total body surface area.[1] The development of improved burn resuscitation, with the well-known endpoints of hematocrit, urine output, and physical signs of euvolemia was hastened by the adjunctive use of blood volume measurement using labeled red cells. Once the patient's blood volume was near normal, excision of the burn wound became feasible. In 1960, Jackson et al. reported excisions up to 35% of the total body surface area, within the first few days after burn injury, bequeathing to their fellow surgeons both an improved method of burn treatment and a model for the ethical, scientific study of progressive surgical interventions. This report can be viewed as a surgical analogue to a Phase-1 study, reporting early excision under defined circumstances as safe and tolerable by burned patients. Their rationale was that burn survival was inversely related to burn size,[2] and their ultimate aim was to determine whether an intervention to rapidly reduce the size of the burn wound could reduce mortality. To this end, they noted that early gains in wound closure were often forfeit in the form of late graft loss, leaving length of stay and overall mortality similar between the groups. The authors also appreciated the importance of infections as a cause of late graft loss and report incidence of positive blood cultures, although no clear differences were appreciated between the early excision and control groups. Finally, from the initial resuscitation through their analysis of mortality, the authors appreciate one of the unseen antagonists of the burned patient: the anemia of thermal burns.[3] In this, the authors were ahead of their time in their appreciation of the contribution of this oft-ignored multifactorial problem to untoward outcomes in burned patients.

REFERENCES

1. Cope O, Langohr JL, Moore FD, Webster RC. Expeditious care of full-thickness burn wounds by surgical excision and grafting. *Ann Surg*. 1947; 125(1): 1–22.
2. Bull JP, Squire JR. A study of mortality in a burns unit: Standards for the evaluation of alternative methods of treatment. *Ann Surg*. 1949; 130(2): 160–173.
3. Moore FD, Peacock WC, Blakely E, Cope O. The anemia of thermal burns. *Ann Surg*. 1946; 124(5): 811–839.

Expert Commentary by Nicholas Namias

The modern history of burn care can be traced back to the story of the Cocoanut Grove fire in Boston in 1942, where there were nearly 1,000 patients with burns and/or smoke inhalation. Experience in burn care in Boston around this fire, while it signaled the first semblance of organized burn care, also signaled the end of the fatalistic approach to burns. The history of burns, up to that time, and the recognition that the status quo could not persist, led to the development of specialized burn centers, and the commitment of the nascent US Army Institute of Surgical Research to make burns a focus of its medical research.

In those days, prior to our modern era, burn patients could be found in the hospital by the odor emanating from the suppuration of burn wounds until the eschars sloughed, with the lucky survivors healing by contraction or delayed grafting. Advances in transfusion and in the understanding of shock, metabolism, infection, and wound healing set the stage for "Primary Excision and Grafting of Large Burns" by Jackson et al.

The modern burn surgeon reading this paper will probably have thought of many of the same questions the authors did (I certainly have), and is still waiting for the definitive randomized controlled trials to settle the safe timing and extent of operation for burn closure. Instead, we operate on the basis of lesser studies, cumulative experience, and wisdom, with this paper acting as the modern foundation for early excision and closure. It led to the next major revolution in 1970, when Janzekovic published "A New Concept in the Early Excision and Immediate Grafting of Burns," which marked the pivot to tangential excision, rather than full thickness excision, and its improved cosmetic and functional outcomes.

Reading Jackson's paper, Janzekovic's later paper, and the firsthand experience of the Cocoanut Grove fire in the autobiography of Francis D. Moore is fundamental to understanding the modern care of burns and advancing, rather the repeating the past mistakes, in burn care.

Editor Notes: This was the seminal work that suggested early excision and grafting of 20%–30% TBSA of deep burns was feasible. The authors randomized 24 patients under 55 years of age to receive early excision and grafting of their full thickness burns, versus waiting 2 to 3 weeks for grafting (standard at the time, 1955–1957). While these authors were unable to demonstrate any real advantages of early excision in their small study, it set the stage for subsequent work that clearly supported this management technique that is the standard of care today.

Limitations:

Small clinical trial;
Limited to a younger population;
No clinician blinding;
No real outcome differences.

CHAPTER 37

Splenic Trauma in Children

Upadhyaya P, Simpson JS. Surg Gynecol Obstet 126(4):781–790, 1968

Expert Commentary by Mitchell Price

The concept of nonoperative management of blunt splenic injury in hemodynamically stable children was first introduced by the Hospital for Sick Children in Toronto, and Upadhyaya's paper is the first reported series of children managed nonoperatively for blunt splenic injury in that institution. Upadhyaya noted that children with splenic injury presented with different signs, symptoms, and prognosis than that of adults. He analyzed 52 children with a diagnosis of splenic rupture from 1956 to 1965. He divided them into three groups with 40 patients undergoing laparotomy and 12 patients being treated nonoperatively. In his study, none of the patients with isolated splenic rupture had signs or symptoms of severe blood loss, no patients had delayed splenic rupture, and there were no mortalities in this group (only those with associated injuries). On laparotomy, a vast majority of patients with splenic rupture did not have active bleeding from their splenic injuries and all lacerations were transverse (not longitudinal) extending from the capsule radially to the hilum. Upadhyaya theorized that indirect blunt trauma produced a transverse rupture, which is dictated by the internal anatomy of the spleen that includes transverse trabeculae and a segmental blood supply. Therefore, a transverse crack, versus a longitudinal laceration, falls along planes that parallel this architecture and can technically reduce the bleeding potential. Other aspects of the spleen in young children include an increase in capsular thickness and less parenchymal bulk with less intracapsular tension, as well as the vascular arrangements, which favor internal shunts that change intrasplenic blood flow, limiting splenic bleeding and hastening clot formation. His conclusion was that minor contusions of the spleen spontaneously stopped bleeding due to the parameters noted above, and if clinical signs resolved in 2–4 hours postinjury, then conservative management without laparotomy can be accomplished successfully. If symptoms warrant, a delayed laparotomy can be done without any increase in morbidity or mortality.

At the time of this article, the accepted management of blunt splenic injury in children consisted of splenectomy with only a selected few individuals doing partial splenectomy or repair. Nonoperative management was considered heresy, based on concerns for increased morbidity and mortality, increase transfusion requirements with its inherent risks, and delayed risk of splenic bleeding.[1] The Hospital for Sick Children in Toronto, and several other institutions championed this nonoperative approach over the ensuing 10–20 years. They collected data demonstrating the efficacy and safety of nonoperative management by showing a decrease in morbidity, mortality, transfusion requirements, and a very low incidence of delayed splenic rupture.[2-5] Another important factor supporting the case for non-management, unbeknownst to Upadhyaya and his colleagues in 1968, was that a couple of years after Upadhyaya's paper, Singer documented the dramatic increased risk for overwhelming, post splenectomy sepsis in children after splenectomy.[6] These factors all helped convince the pediatric surgical community that nonoperative management was safe and effective, but, at that time, the practice of nonoperative management was not standardized or validated. It wasn't until Stylianos and the American Pediatric Surgery Association (APSA) published a landmark study in 2000,[7] that a specific set of consensus guidelines were delineated. These evidence-based guidelines concerned the grade-based need for intensive care observation, length of stay in the hospital, routine imaging, and activity restrictions after discharge. Presently, the standard of care for splenic rupture in a hemodynamically stable child is nonoperative management, and this has spread to the adult population.[8] This dramatic reversal in management was pioneered by Upadhyaya and his colleagues in Toronto some 50 years ago. An excellent review article on this subject by Upadhyaya, himself, is worthwhile reading and has been included in the bibliography.[9]

REFERENCES

1. Davies DA, Pearl RH, Ein SH, et al. Management of blunt splenic injury in children: Evolution of the nonoperative approach. *J Pediatr Surg.* 2009; 44: 1005–1008.
2. Ein SH, Shandling B, Simpson JS, et al. Nonoperative management of traumatized spleen in children: How and why. *J Pediatr Surg.* 1978; 13: 117–119.
3. Pearl RH, Wesson DE, Spence LJ, et al. Splenic Injury: A 5 year update with improved results and changing criteria for conservative management. *J Pediatr Surg.* 1989; 24: 428–431.
4. Sjovall A, Hirsch K. Blunt abdominal trauma in children: Risks of nonoperative treatment. *J Pediatr Surg.* 1977; 32: 1169–1174.
5. Lally KP, Rosario V, Mahour GH, Wolley MM. Evolution in the management of splenic injury in children. *Surg Gynec Obstet.* 1990; 170: 245–248. Review.
6. Singer DB. Postsplenectomy sepsis. *Perspect Pediatr Pathol.* 1973; 1: 285–311. Review.
7. Stylianos SS. Evidence based guidelines for resource utilization in children with isolated spleen or liver injury: The APSA Trauma Committee. *J Pediatr Surg.* 2000; 35: 164–169.
8. Cogbill TH, Moore EE, Jurkovich GJ, et al. Nonoperative management of blunt splenic trauma: A multicenter experience. *J Trauma.* 1989: 29: 1312–1317.
9. Upadhyaya P. Conservative management of splenic trauma: History and current trends. *Pediatr Surg Int.* 2003; 19(9–10): 617–627.

Expert Commentary by Andrew B. Peitzman

A paradigm shift in the management of blunt injury to solid organs, in this case the spleen, has been remarkable. The incidence of overwhelming post-splenectomy infections (OPSIs) in infants and the observation that healed spleens were found at autopsy led the pediatric surgeons to initiate the effort to preserve the injured spleen. The Upadhyaya paper is a report of 52 children with splenic injury, a third of whom were managed nonoperatively. Even in the patients undergoing splenectomy, the majority of the spleens had stopped bleeding. Realize that this paper was published prior to the availability of computed tomography (CT). The promulgation of CT has allowed nonoperative management of solid organs to become standard. Furthermore, even in 1968, the authors commented about differences in injury pattern and quantity of hemoperitoneum in adults versus children. Essentially all children with blunt injury to the spleen stable enough for CT can be successfully observed.

The decision making and natural history of blunt injury to the spleen (BSI) in adults is more complicated, and the focus of the remaining discussion. The seminal papers from the Eastern Association for the Surgery of Trauma (EAST) documented the failure rate for nonoperative management (NOM) of blunt splenic injury in adults as 10.8%. The risk of failure of NOM increased with age, Injury Severity Score (ISS), grade of splenic injury, and quantity of hemoperitoneum. Eighty percent of splenic injury was grade 1–3, generally, safely observed. However, one-half of grade 4 and over 90% of grade 5 splenic injuries went directly to the operating room. Ultimately, 98% of grade 5 splenic injury underwent laparotomy. Importantly, assessment of the outcome of failed NOM management revealed a 12% mortality, 60% of which were preventable deaths.

Studies utilizing the National Trauma Data Bank (NTDB) confirmed a failure rate of over 50% for grade 4 and 5 splenic injury. A more recent study of grades 4 and 5 using Trauma Quality Improvement Project (TQIP) reported a failure of NOM in 18% of grade 4 injury and 29% of grade 5. However, 65% of grade 5 injuries underwent immediate splenectomy. Thus, 78% of grade 5 splenic injuries ultimately underwent laparotomy. Thus, it is uncommon that a grade 5 injury can be observed, with a high failure rate with observation alone. NOM of grade 4 splenic injury is more reasonable if the patient is stable.

The role of angiography/embolization (AE) in management of blunt splenic injury is still in evolution. The patient with active extravasation or pseudoaneurysm on CT should undergo AE. Recent papers suggest that empiric angioembolization for grade 4 or 5 BSI, even without extravasation or pseudoaneurysm on CT or angiography, significantly decreases the incidence of failure of NOM. This is our practice.

In a recent survey, it was reported that 85% of trauma surgeons do not reimage BSI with CT. However, we do obtain a follow-up CT for grades 3–5 BSI based on several papers that report a doubling of pseudoaneurysms found with this protocol.

Last, subcapsular hematomas (SCH) of the spleen remain problematic. A report from 2015 found subcapsular splenic hematomas in 13% of patients undergoing NOM. The failure rate of NOM was 1.5% in patients without SCH and 35.3% in patients with SCH. The authors reported that only grade of splenic injury and presence of SCH predicted failure of NOM.

Editor Notes: This was the first large case series of children with splenic injuries managed without laparotomy. Twelve of the 52 patients with trauma to the left upper quadrant of the abdomen were observed despite signs and symptoms of splenic rupture. At the time, splenectomy was considered the only option for these patients. Subsequent work in both children and adults led to a radical reversal in management of these patients. For example, rather than 85% undergoing laparotomy, with 50% splenectomy as was noted in the late 1980s, today only about 25% of patients with splenic injury undergo abdominal exploration.

Limitations:

Retrospective review;
Small number of patients;
The diagnosis of splenic injury may have been incorrect as the study was performed prior to the advent of CT scanning;
There is limited information on the clinical course of these children who were not operated upon.

CHAPTER 38

Status of Nonoperative Management of Blunt Hepatic Injuries in 1995: A Multicenter Experience with 404 Patients

Pachter HL, Knudson MM, Esrig B, Ross S, Hoyt D, Cogbill T, Sherman H, Scalea T, Harrison P, Shackford S, et al. J Trauma 40(1):31–38, 1996

Abstract   Nonoperative management is presently considered the treatment modality of choice in over 50% of adult patients sustaining blunt hepatic trauma who meet inclusion criteria. A multicenter study was retrospectively undertaken to assess whether the combined experiences at level I trauma centers could validate the currently reported high success rate, low morbidity, and virtually nonexistent mortality associated with this approach. Thirteen level I trauma centers accrued 404 adult patients sustaining blunt hepatic injuries managed nonoperatively over the last 5 years. Seventy-two percent of the injuries resulted from motor vehicle crashes. The mean injury severity score for the entire group was 20.2 (range, 4–75), and the American Association for the Surgery of Trauma computerized axial tomography scan grading was as follows: grade I, 19% ($n = 76$); grade II, 31% ($n = 124$); grade III, 36 ($n = 146$); grade IV, 10% ($n = 42$); and grade V, 4% ($n = 16$). There were 27 deaths (7%) in the series, with 59% directly related to head trauma. Only two deaths (0.4%) could be attributed to hepatic injury. Twenty-one (5%) complications were documented, with the most common being hemorrhage, occurring in 14 (3.5%). Only 3 (0.7%) of these 14 patients required surgical intervention, 6 were treated by transfusions alone (0.5 to 5 U), 4 underwent angioembolization, and 1 was further observed. Other complications included 2 bilomas and 3 perihepatic abscesses (all drained percutaneously). Two small bowel injuries were initially missed (0.5%) and diagnosed 2 and 3 days after admission. Overall, 6 patients required operative intervention: 3 for hemorrhage, 2 for missed enteric injuries, and 1 for persistent sepsis after unsuccessful percutaneous drainage. Average length of stay was 13 days. Nonoperative management of blunt hepatic injuries is clearly the treatment modality of choice in hemodynamically stable patients, irrespective of grade of injury or degree of hemoperitoneum. Current data would suggest that 50%–80% (47% in this series) of all adult patients with blunt hepatic injuries are candidates for this form of therapy. Exactly 98.5% of patients analyzed in this study successfully avoided operative intervention. Bleeding complications are infrequently encountered (3.5%) and can often be managed nonoperatively. Although grades IV and V injuries composed 14% of the series, they represented 66.6% of the patients requiring operative intervention and thus merit constant re-evaluation and close observation in critical care units. The optimal time for follow-up computerized axial tomography scanning seems to be within 7–10 days after injury.

Author Commentary by H. Leon Pachter

We often take for granted approaches to surgical problems that currently are the standard of care without reflecting on the growing pains so inherent during their gestational period. Nonoperative management of blunt hepatic injuries, when criteria are met, is universally accepted as the gold standard of care. But it wasn't always that way. In the late 1970s, when I presented the first case of non-operative management of a blunt hepatic injury at Bellevue Hospital, I felt like a bad Shakespearian actor being pelted with rotten fruit. Senior faculty smirked and expounded out loud "You did what?"

They were not alone in their skepticism as they were joined by the glitterati and illuminati of Trauma Surgery in their rebuke, which more often than not, they espoused in the "absolute," and emphatic hyperbole. In 1977, one of these luminaries in an article published in the *Annals of Surgery* noted that "the structure and consistency of liver tissue is unsuitable for spontaneous hemostasis following parenchymal disruption." Reading between the lines, the concept of nonoperative management of blunt hepatic injuries was, at best, not possible, and at worst downright dangerous. This philosophy continued to be perpetuated on the surgical world even into the early 1990s, despite several publications attesting to the safety and efficacy of this approach. Challenges to accepted principles established as "sacred cows" in surgical management are usually not met with unbridled enthusiasm as change, in any walk of life, makes people uneasy and uncomfortable. In 1990, another trauma luminary felt compelled to voice his concern about the appropriateness of the non-operative management of blunt hepatic injuries. His stated concerns regarding this approach revolved around two key factors: (1) missed associated injuries, and (2) significant ongoing blood loss. In his opinion, it was "… prudent to operate early," and thus avoid missed enteric injuries while keeping blood loss to a minimum.

Broken down into its essence, the hesitancy in routinely accepting a nonopera-tive approach to blunt hepatic injuries were as follows:

1. What percent of patients are candidates for this approach?
2. Which classification of hepatic injury is this approach safe?
3. How much hemoperitoneum is acceptable?
4. Does this approach require excessive blood transfusions?
5. How often is it successful?
6. What percentage of enteric injuries are missed?

Between 1988 and 1995, I accrued from the literature 495 adult patients from 14 institutions with blunt injuries managed nonoperatively. Collectively, they achieved a 94% success rate with minimal transfusions, complications, and ongoing hemorrhagic rates. Most importantly, there were no missed enteric injuries.

In order to both see if these results were reproducible and to answer the aforementioned hesitancy questions, we embarked on a 13 level I trauma centers multi-institutional study encompassing 404 patients over a 5-year period.

This paper established nonoperative management of blunt hepatic injuries, in the hemodynamically stable patient, as the treatment modality of choice. The credence factor, which lends to the veracity of the results, is that the data emanated from 13 well-respected level I trauma centers in the United States.

At the time of the writing, nearly 50% of adult patients were candidates for this approach, and 98.5% avoided surgical intervention. Current data would suggest that, perhaps, 75%–80% of patients may be candidates for this approach. There were only 2 related hepatic injury deaths (0.4%). It would appear that any grade of hepatic injury I–V, if meeting criteria, can be managed nonoperatively. However, it is worth noting that 66% of the failures in this study were classified as grade IV–V. Clearly, these patients require very close observation. However, newer techniques in "stenting" vascular injuries and advances in angioembolization may increase the number of these patients that can avoid surgery.

The intent of this approach is to avoid unnecessary and often complicated hepatic surgery and transfusion rates. This paper showed that even a 500-cc hemoperitoneum, in the face of hemodynamic stability, can be managed nonoperatively.

The incidence of missed enteric injuries, one percent in this study, and 3% reported elsewhere is a series concern. However, with close observation and prompt surgical intervention no patient suffered any untoward result.

No approach is perfect to any injury, but we should not be hampered by tactics that worked in the past but may not be as relevant today as they had been. This paper established nonoperative management of blunt hepatic injuries as the preferred approach based on data from highly reliable sources.

REFERENCES

Flint LM, Mays ET, Aaron WS, et al. Selectivity in management of hepatic trauma. *Ann Surg.* 1977; 185: 613–618.

Hiatt JR, Harrier HD, Koenig BV, et al. Nonoperative management of major blunt liver trauma with hemoperitoneum. *Arch of Surg.* 1990; 125: 101.

Pachter HL, Hofstetter SR. The current status of nonoperative management of adult blunt hepatic injuries. *Am J Surg.* 1995; 169: 442.

Trunkey D. Blunt hepatic trauma nonoperative management in adults: Invited commentary. *Arch Surg.* 1990; 125: 909.

Expert Commentary by Bellal A. Joseph

Liver injuries have always been one of the most difficult to manage and have puzzled trauma surgeons for decades. Management of liver injuries has evolved in the past 30 years. The single greatest advancement has been the evolution of nonoperative management of liver injuries. In the early 1970s, more than 80% of the liver injuries were managed operatively. In the late 1990s, 80%–90% of these injuries were successfully managed by the nonoperative approach. This changing pattern in the management of complex hepatic injuries, which has been referred to as a paradigm shift, is attributed to the advancement of imaging and minimally invasive technologies.

This landmark paper defined the multimodal approach for the management of liver injuries some 30 years ago, most of which are still utilized today. It laid the cornerstone for the nonoperative management of patients with liver injuries, who are hemodynamically stable, and paved the way for the nonoperative management utilizing interventional radiology. Currently, we have expanded the conservative management of liver injuries even to a subset of hemodynamically unstable patients who respond to initial resuscitation. This has been made possible due to revolutionizing advancements in resuscitation strategies, improved sensitivity of diagnostic modalities, and the growth of interventional medicine through minimally invasive angioembolization techniques. The technique of angioembolization has been incorporated at different time points of patient care, which has a significant impact on survival of patients with liver injuries. For instance, angioembolization can be utilized as an adjunct to packing in patients where hemostasis cannot be achieved with packing alone. The more recent availability of intraoperative angiographic capabilities has made this decision easier, and embolization can be performed in the surgical theatre.

Some of the surgical techniques described in this paper have survived the test of time and are still critical to achieving hemostasis in patients with complex liver injuries. These include the use of portal triad occlusion (Pringle maneuver) and the finger fracture technique. Over time, we have learned that direct suture ligation of the parenchymal bleeding vessel, perihepatic packing, repair of venous injury under total vascular isolation, and damage control surgery with the utilization of preoperative and/or postoperative angioembolization are the preferred methods, compared to anatomical resection of the liver and use of the atriocaval shunt. In addition, a better understanding of the pathophysiology of liver trauma has allowed us to move from a prolonged continuous occlusion of the portal triad to a shorter intermittent clamping leading to improved liver ischemia tolerance.

Liver injuries are diverse, complex, and still highly lethal. A trauma surgeon should possess not only an arsenal of surgical techniques, but also the capacity to decide when to operate and when to hold back. The principle *"Putting brain in gear before knife in motion"* holds true here. The ultimate decision for operative intervention must be based on the available resources and hemodynamic status of the patient. The multimodal approach to liver injuries and the utilization of minimally invasive techniques have led to better solutions for unfolding this puzzle.

Editor Notes: While not the first study to describe the success of nonoperative management of liver trauma, this huge retrospective study clearly established observation as the cornerstone of management of hemodynamically stable patients with imaging-proven injuries, irrespective of severity of injury. Only 14 of 404 (5%) patients managed nonoperatively developed hepatic complications, and just 6 required operative intervention (typically from high-grade lesions).

Limitations:

Likely selection bias pushing marginal patients to surgery could have possibility that some complications may not have been reported.

CHAPTER 39

Gunshot Wound of the Abdomen: Role of Selective Conservative Management

Demetriades D, Charalambides D, Lakhoo M, Pantanowitz D.
Br J Surg 78(2):220–222, 1991

Abstract This prospective study includes 146 patients with gunshot wounds of the abdomen. One hundred five patients (72%) had an acute abdomen on admission and were operated on immediately. The remaining 41 patients (28%) had minimal or equivocal abdominal signs and were observed with serial clinical examinations. Seven of the observed patients needed subsequent laparotomy, but there was no mortality or serious morbidity. Had a policy of mandatory exploration for abdominal gunshot wound been applied, the incidence of unnecessary or negative laparotomies would have been 27%. By using a policy of selective conservatism, this figure was only 5%. We suggest that abdominal gunshot wounds should be assessed and managed exactly like knife wounds. Physical examination is reliable in detecting significant intra-abdominal injuries. Many carefully selected patients with abdominal gunshot wounds can safely be managed nonoperatively.

Author Commentary by Demetrios Demetriades

Surgical dogma often dominates many practices in trauma surgery. Statements like "this is what I was taught, this is what I teach" or "it is in the textbooks" or "this has been the standard of care for decades" are common and often perpetuate practices that have no scientific basis. A classic example of surgical dogma is the history of the management of gunshot wounds (GSWs) to the abdomen. For many decades, mandatory laparotomy was the standard of care for all abdominal GSWs. The medical literature in the 1980s or 1990s is dominated by statements such as "No attempt is made to identify a specific indication for laparotomy other than the presence of a gunshot wound that appears to have penetrated the abdominal cavity" or "Laparotomy should be performed regardless of physical examination or estimated trajectory." However, many studies consistently showed that 20%–30% of laparotomies for abdominal GSWs were nontherapeutic! Other studies reported that nontherapeutic laparotomies were associated with a high incidence of complications.

The concept of mandatory laparotomy was first challenged by South African centers with large volumes of GSWs. Many patients with GSWs to the abdomen were completely asymptomatic, and, as part of the triage system, other patients with hemodynamic instability or peritonitis were prioritized for the operative room! Many hours after admission we would find it difficult to operate on an asymptomatic patient! This was the birth of the selective nonoperative management (SNOM) of abdominal GSWs!

In 1991, we prepared a manuscript describing our experience with this approach. It was a prospective study of 146 patients with abdominal GSWs, and 23% of these cases were successfully managed nonoperatively. We concluded that SNOM for abdominal GSWs was a safe option. *The manuscript was rejected by numerous journals and some of the reviewers were openly hostile and dismissive!* The manuscript was accepted and published by the *British Journal of Surgery* in 1991.

The study was largely ignored by US trauma centers. In the mid-1990s, there were the first reports in the US literature of a small number of patients with GSWs to the right thoracoabdominal area treated nonoperatively (Renz and Feliciano, *J Trauma*, 1994, and Chvielewski, *Am Surg*, 1995), but mandatory exploration remained the standard of care.

In 1993, I was recruited as the trauma director at the LAC+USC medical center, one of the largest trauma centers in the country. With the help of Dr. George Velmahos, another South African-trained surgeon, we systematically introduced the practice of selective nonoperative management. This was considered heresy, at the time, and I had major hesitations in submitting for publication a completed prospective study. I was encouraged to submit the manuscript for publication in the *Archives of Surgery* by a 1996 editorial by Nance ML and Nance FC in the *Journal of Trauma*, with the title "It Is Time We Told the Emperor about His Clothes." The editorial stated that "The time has come to challenge a philosophy that accepts an unnecessary laparotomy in at least 20% of subjects. Selective nonoperative management should be used for GSWs as it is already being used in patients with blunt trauma or stab wounds." In the next few years, the USC group published numerous studies that demonstrated the safety and cost-effectiveness of selective nonoperative management of GSWs to the anterior and posterior abdomen and solid abdominal organs. This practice has now become the new standard of care in many trauma centers. In a 2011 study (Jansen et al., *Injury*, 2011), 74% of US surgeons practiced selective nonoperative management of abdominal GSWs. In recent TQIP studies, 34.5% of 5,411 isolated GSWs to the liver and 29.2% of isolated GSWs to the kidney were managed nonoperatively.

Expert Commentary by David V. Feliciano

With the advent of trauma centers and patient management protocols in the United States in the 1960s and 1970s, one of the major principles of care was "don't miss an injury." This was based on the fact that most of the injuries encountered on a routine cervical exploration, sternotomy or thoracotomy, or laparotomy could be readily repaired with suture or resection by a well-trained general surgeon. But missing an injury acutely to the cervical or thoracic esophagus, a mediastinal vessel, the heart, or the retroperitoneal duodenum or colon would be lethal for 25%–100% of the patients.

This prompted mandatory cervical explorations for stab or gunshot wounds penetrating the platysma muscle of the neck, mandatory mediastinal exploration for presumed mediastinal traverse by a missile, and mandatory laparotomies for anterior or flank stab wounds presumed to penetrate the peritoneal cavity and all gunshot wounds in proximity to the abdomen (including the thoracoabdomen, flank, and back). At one level I trauma center in the 1980s, the "mandatory operation" policy resulted in the following annually: 25–30 negative or nontherapeutic cervical explorations, 3–7 negative mediastinal explorations, 75–80 negative laparotomies for abdominal stab wounds, and 10 negative laparotomies for abdominal gunshot wounds. Reviewing the literature from the 1960s to the 1990s, a mandatory operative approach resulted in a 25%–40% negative or nontherapeutic laparotomy rate for patients with blunt abdominal trauma or presumed penetrating anterior or flank stab wounds and a 15%–27% rate for patients with gunshot wounds of the abdomen. In patients with penetrating wounds of the flank or back, especially gunshot wounds, the negative or nontherapeutic laparotomy rate was an incredible 70%–85%. And, over time, the morbidity of a negative or nontherapeutic laparotomy became well-known in all level I trauma centers.

The logical response to the newly recognized problem of unnecessary laparotomies after penetrating trauma was a more selective approach pioneered by Gerry Shaftan and Carter Nance for patients with abdominal stab wounds in the 1960s. The major contribution of Demetriades et al. was the recognition that many missile wounds in proximity to the abdomen do not penetrate. Currently, this is presumed to be from victims turning away from assailants holding a handgun and from the obese abdominal walls of many victims in the United States. And, there will always be a 2%–5% group of "lucky" patients in whom the peritoneal cavity or retroperitoneum is violated, but the oblique intraperitoneal or retroperitoneal track (anterior or posterior-to-flank or flank-to-anterior or posterior) of the missile misses all hollow viscera and doesn't cause enough hepatic or renal damage to prompt a laparotomy. The other valuable message from Demetriades et al. reiterates that of Shaftan and Nance. A low velocity, low kinetic energy penetrating missile wound of the abdomen is not all that dissimilar from a stab wound; that is, in the small subset of asymptomatic or modestly symptomatic patients who are hemodynamically stable, serial physical examinations are an acceptable form of initial management rather than a mandatory laparotomy.

Editor Notes: This manuscript reported on 41 of 146 patients (28%) with penetrating abdominal wounds who were minimally symptomatic and underwent careful observation. Only 7/41 of these patients went on to exploration without mortality or serious morbidity. Prior to this time, gunshot wounds to the abdomen underwent mandatory laparotomy, even if completely asymptomatic. This paper and other similar studies led to our current selective management of penetrating wounds.

Limitations:

Small population;
Unclear frequency of serial exams and expertise of the examiner;
Uncertain outpatient follow-up process.

CHAPTER 40

Pelvic Fracture in Multiple Trauma: Classification by Mechanism Is Key to Pattern of Organ Injury, Resuscitative Requirements, and Outcome

Dalal SA, Burgess AR, Siegel JH, Young JW, Brumback RJ, Poka A, Dunham CM, Gens D, Bathon H. J Trauma 29(7):981–1000; discussion 1000–1002, 1989

Abstract   Three hundred forty-three multiple trauma patients with major pelvic ring disruption were studied and subdivided into four major groups by mechanism of injury: antero-posterior compression (APC), lateral compression (LC), vertical shear (VS), and combined mechanical injury (CMI). Acetabular fractures that did not disrupt the pelvic ring were excluded. The mode of injury was: MVA, 57.4%; motorcycle, 9.3%; fall, 9.3%; pedestrian, 17.8%; crush, 3.8%. The LC and APC groups were divided into grades 1–3 of increasing severity. The pattern of organ injury: including brain, lung, liver, spleen, bowel, bladder, pelvic vascular injury (PVASI), retroperitoneal hematoma (RPH), and complications: circulatory shock, sepsis, ARDS, abnormal physiology, and 24-hour total fluid volume administration were all evaluated as a function of mortality (M). As the LC grade increased from 1 to 3, there was increased % incidence of PVASI, RPH, shock, and 24-hour volume needs. However, the large incidence of brain, lung, and upper abdominal visceral injuries as causes of death in grade 1 and 2 fell in LC3, with limitation of the LC3 injury pattern to the pelvis. As APC grade increased from 1 to 3, there was increased % injury to spleen, liver, bowel, PVASI with RPH, shock, sepsis, and ARDS, and large increases in volume needs, with important incidence of brain and lung injuries in all grades. Organ injury patterns and % M associated with vertical shear were similar to those with severe grades of APC, but CMI had an associated organ injury pattern similar to lower grades of APC and LC fractures. The pattern of injury in APC3 was correlated with the greatest 24-hour fluid requirements and with a rise in mortality as the APC grade rose. However, there were major differences in the causes of death in LC versus APC injuries, with brain injury compounded by shock being significant contributors in LC. In contrast, in APC there were significant influences of shock, sepsis, and ARDS related to the massive torso forces delivered in APC, with large volume losses from visceral organs and pelvis of greater influence in APC, but brain injury was not a significant cause of death. These data indicate that the mechanical force type and severity of the pelvic fracture are the keys to the expected organ injury pattern, resuscitation needs, and mortality.

Author Commentary by Andrew R. Burgess

The "thought and inspiration" for our 1989 article, originated in an institution unique for the period.[1] The authors were full-time general and orthopedic trauma staff, most fellowship-trained. The layout/protocols of the 1980s Shock-Trauma Center produced: (1) resuscitation area in continuity with Trauma ORs, (2) attending surgeons having rapid access to patients and EMS providers, and (3) 75% of patients admitted from scene. Evaluation was based on vital signs, physical exam, plain radiographs, and lab values.

Simultaneously, intuitional interest was growing in crash research.

In 1980, Pennal and Tile had published "Arriving at a Logical Classification of Pelvic Injury."[2] "The Anterior and Lateral Compression types, while very different, each have stable and unstable subtypes associated with them. Vertical Shear type is always unstable."

Young and Burgess reviewed musculoskeletal radiographs, were often aware of scene conditions, and sub-classified pelvic disruption, based on Pennal-Tile's classification.[3] They considered observed severity/direction of impact, noting radiographic signs of direction *and* degree of deforming force.

We approached data from two points: Did vector and amplitude of the injurious force to the pelvis cause predictable patterns of associated injury (viscera, CNS, etc.) and later, could patterns seen on plain films be correlated with the direction/velocity of impact? Acetabular fractures were included, essentially, as a control.

Many clinical impressions were born out by the data.

In spite of major changes in vehicle occupant protection and seat belt compliance (from 10% to 90%) since written, some factors deserve notice: APC III fracture types, both in 1990[6] and 2017, still result in the most severe hemorrhage (and in 2017 need "hemorrhage control");[7] LC I pelvic fractures in the elderly have more hemorrhage in younger patients,[8,9] perhaps due to plaque "stiffening" of the internal iliac watershed.

I remained interested in pelvic fractures, both in early management in poly-traumatized patients and in related crash mechanism research (CIREN). Although the patients in our 1989 article were injured by varied mechanisms, such as MVA (57%), pedestrian, motorcycle, and crush, detailed *automotive* crash reconstruction[4,11–14] taught a significant amount about *all* mechanisms, since the musculoskeletal injuries of such patients are often quite descriptive in the context of known PDOF (Principle Direction of Force) and ΔV (change in velocity). As work continued, applying the common classifications to treatment protocols yielded good results, some findings of hemorrhage in APC III[6] were duplicated as recently as this year.[7] Increased hemorrhage in early versus recent work dealing with classification and mechanism issues are presented as "blood loss" or need for transfused blood products in the earlier works, while more recent literature presents the same risk issues (mechanism and/or age) as requiring interventional angiographic hemorrhage control.

Findings in two studies, 26 years apart (see above), described the same issues, differing primarily in the titles of the articles, one presented as "Effective Classification System and Treatment Protocols" (1990), the other being, "Pelvic Fracture Pattern Predicts the Need for Hemorrhage Control Intervention ..." The first article found that APC III averaged 35 units of blood replacement in 48 hours, the second article found 83% of APC II injuries required hemorrhage control intervention. The second re-emphasizes findings of 26 years earlier.

For reasons above, I strongly believe an early AP pelvis film is still required, especially in a high energy event or in a patient in extremis. I consider it a "vital sign" to experienced trauma docs who should recognize the high-risk type of pelvic ring destruction and rapidly upshift the aggressiveness of their resuscitation/work-up/intervention.

Early placement of immobilization (binder, sheet, exfix) of high energy, skeletally unstable pelvis has value in (1) elevating systolic BP, (2) reducing hemorrhage, and (3) reducing risk of transport.

Studying *mechanism–dependent* pelvic fractures: vehicle occupant; motorcycle; pedestrian; falls; crush; and so on, yields valuable data, and certain fracture patterns are predictably common to certain mechanisms: LC III to crush, vertical shear to falls, APC III to motorcycles, LCI to "T-bone" MVA, and studying fractures by known mechanism provides valuable data from Stein[11] and Eastridge.[5]

Expert Commentary by Clifford B. Jones

The authors determined how the injury force, magnitude, and direction impacted the pelvic ring and associated organ injuries. The initial patient evaluation consisted of the physical exam, vitals, pelvic ring X-ray, and EMS account of accident scene. Since no routine CT exams were obtained, the initial AP pelvic ring X-ray became another vital sign in the injured patient assessment. Early crash test research was correlated with mechanism and injuries. Therefore, MVA "T-bone" had a LC1. MCA hit from the front had an APC. Crush injury had LC3. A pedestrian run over had ipsilateral LC and a contralateral AP, the bilateral injury described as LC3. Fall had an ipsilateral VS. The nomenclature (LC, APC, VS, and CMI) now became common and consistent vocabulary for the orthopaedic, trauma, and radiology teams.

The authors then determined how the initial pelvic ring X-ray could predict organ injury pattern, associated complications, and death in polytrauma patients. LC were usually hemodynamically stable, but when hypotensive, the usual etiology was solid organ injury and aortic injuries. Increasing grade of LC from 1 to 3 had a higher incidence of brain, lung, and visceral injuries. The causes of death were brain injury compounded by shock. APC injury increased from 1 to 3, higher incidence of spleen, liver, bowel, vascular, retroperitoneal hematoma injuries were noted. Therefore, increasing APC had increasing volume resuscitation needs, shock, sepsis, and ARDS as causes of death but not brain injury. VS was similar to higher grades LC. CMI was similar to higher grades APC but organ injury similar to lower LC and APC. Injury or accident force vector and magnitude could be extrapolated from the pelvic injury X-ray. This landmark publication impacted clinical practice with the ability to correlate the initial pelvic picture with expected organ injury pattern, resuscitation needs, angiography assistance, and mortality. From this groundbreaking work and injury pattern analysis, the crash injury research center (NHTSA) originated and blossomed being able to determine delta velocity change and vector, principal direction of force (PDOF) in predicting injury and patterns.

Modern pelvic injury assessment differs from the study population. Pelvic binders are utilized liberally in the field applied by EMS or in the trauma bay, especially in hemodynamically unstable patients. Pelvic binders are advantageous, reducing pelvic volume and enhancing resuscitation. Trauma patients are assessed in a binder with a CT scan prior to or in substitution of an initial pelvic X-ray. The injury CT is then reformatted with 3-D reconstruction, which obviates traditional pelvic X-rays. The advantage of this is an initial assessment of solid organ injury, bleeding (blush), and occult pelvic ring injury. The disadvantage of only CT assessment is that one can lose the ability to predict ongoing blood loss source and evolving injury patterns. Communication with the trauma, orthopaedic, and radiology teams is still paramount.

In conclusion, the original pelvic injury picture (now 3-D CT) is very well worth a thousand words in being able to help services communicate, predict organ injury pattern, probable resuscitation, and potential for death.

REFERENCES

1. Dalal SA, Burgess AR, Siegel JH, Young JW, Brumback RJ, et al. Pelvic fracture in multiple trauma: Classification by mechanism is key to pattern of organ injury, resuscitative requirements, and outcome. *J Trauma*. 1989; 29(7): 981–1000; discussion 1000–1002.
2. Pennal GF, Tile M, Waddell JP, Garside H. Pelvic disruption: Assessment and classification. *Clin Orthop Relat Res*. 1980; (151): 12–21.
3. Young JWR, Burgess AR, Brumback RJ. Lateral compression fractures of the pelvis: The importance of plain radiographs in the diagnosis and surgical management. *Skeletal Radiol*. 1986; 15: 103–104.

4. Siegel JH, Dalal SA, Burgess AR, Young JW. Pattern of organ injuries in pelvic fracture: Impact force implications for survival and death in motor vehicle injuries. *Accid Anal Prev.* 1990; 22(5): 457–466.
5. Eastridge BJ, Burgess AR. Pedestrian pelvic fractures: 5-year experience of a major urban trauma center. *J Trauma.* 1997; 42(4): 695–700.
6. Burgess AR, Eastridge BJ, Young JW, et al. Pelvic ring disruptions: Effective classification system and treatment protocols. *J Trauma.* 1990; 30(7): 848–856.
7. Costantini TW, Coimbra R, Holcomb JB, et al. Pelvic fracture pattern predicts the need for hemorrhage control intervention: Results of an AAST multi-institutional study. *J Trauma Acute Care Surg.* 2017; 82(6): 1030–1038.
8. Kimbrell BJ, Valmahos GC, Chan LS, Demetriades D. Angiographic embolization for pelvic fractures in older patients. *Arch Surg.* 2004; 139(7): 728–732; discussion 732–733.
9. Henry SM, Pollak AN, Jones AL, Boswell S, Scalea TM. Pelvic fracture in geriatric patients: A distinct clinical entity. *J Trauma.* 2002; 53(1): 15–20.
10. Furey AJ, O'Toole RV, Nascone JW, et al. Classification of pelvic fractures: Analysis of inter- and intraobserver variability using the Young-Burgess and Tile classification systems. *Orthopedics.* 2009; 32(6): 401.
11. Gokcen EC, Burgess AR, Siegel JH, Mason-Gonzalez S, Dischinger PC, Ho SM. Pelvic fracture mechanism of injury in vehicular trauma patients. *J Trauma.* 1994; 36(6): 789–795; discussion 795–796.
12. Stein DM, O'Connor JV, Kufera JA, et al. Risk factors associated with pelvic fractures sustained in motor vehicle collisions involving newer vehicles. *J Trauma.* 2006; 61(1): 21–30; discussion 30–31.
13. Ryb GE, Dischinger PC, Kufera JA, Burch CA. Delta V, principle direction of force, and restraint use contributions to motor vehicle crash mortality. *J Trauma.* 2007; 63(5): 1000–1005.
14. Dischinger PC, Siegel JH, Ho SM, Kufera JA. Effect of change in velocity on the development of medical complications in patients with multisystem trauma sustained in vehicular crashes. *Accid Anal Prev.* 1998; 30(6): 831–837.

Editor Notes: This landmark study defined pelvic fractures by mechanism. Organ injury patterns, resuscitation needs, and mortality were associated with specific mechanical force type and severity of pelvic injury. Pelvic fracture categories were Anterior Posterior Compression, Lateral Compression, Vertical Shear, combined injuries, and acetabular fractures. The authors found a high incidence of associated brain injury with Anterior Posterior Compression mechanism. In addition, they noted a greater likelihood of shock mandating resuscitation with more fluid and blood products in the most severe pelvic injuries. This classification of pelvic fractures into clinically relevant subtypes helped promote the development of the multimodality and multidisciplinary team approach that we utilize today.

Limitations:

Intervention with skeletal traction and/or angiographic embolization was not protocolized or prioritized;
Rectal and urologic injuries were not specifically described;
Open pelvic fractures were not included in the analysis.

CHAPTER 41

Intra-Abdominal Hypertension after Life-Threatening Penetrating Abdominal Trauma: Prophylaxis, Incidence, and Clinical Relevance to Gastric Mucosal pH and Abdominal Compartment Syndrome

Ivatury RR, Porter JM, Simon RJ, Islam S, John R, Stahl WM. J Trauma 44(6):1016–1021; discussion 1021–1023, 1998

Abstract   The authors studied the relatively novel concept of routine intra-abdominal pressure (IAP) measurements to detect the presence of intra-abdominal hypertension (IAH). They identified, through the use of gastric tonometry and intramucosal gastric pH measurements, that visceral acidosis and ischemia occurred at IAPs that had previously been thought to be clinically insignificant. Further, they noted that failure to intervene in a timely fashion resulted in worsening multisystem organ failure and death. Most importantly, they demonstrated that prophylactic abdominal decompression with maintenance of an open abdomen resulted in significantly improved patient survival and reduced organ failure.

Objective   To define the incidence, prophylaxis, and treatment of intra-abdominal hypertension and its relevance to gut mucosal pH (pHi), multiorgan dysfunction syndrome, and the abdominal compartment syndrome (ACS).

Methods   Seventy patients in the SICU at a level I trauma center (1992–1996) with life-threatening penetrating abdominal trauma had intra-abdominal pressure estimated by bladder pressure. pHi was measured by gastric tonometry every 4–6 hours. IAH (intra-abdominal pressure > 25 cm of H_2O) was treated by bedside or operating room laparotomy.

Results   Injury severity was comparable between patients who had mesh closure as prophylaxis for IAH (n = 45) and those who had fascial suture (n = 25). IAH was seen in 10 (22.2%) in the mesh group versus 13 (52%) in the fascial suture group (p = 0.012) for an overall incidence of 32.9%. Forty-two patients had pHi monitoring and 11 of them had IAH. Of the 11 patients, eight patients (72.7%) had acidotic pHi (7.10 ± 0.2) with IAH without exhibiting the classic signs of ACS. The pHi improved after abdominal decompression in six and none developed ACS. Only two patients with IAH and low pHi went on to develop ACS, despite abdominal decompression. Multiorgan dysfunction syndrome points and death were less in patients without IAH than those with IAH and in patients who had mesh closure.

Conclusions   IAH is frequent after major abdominal trauma. It may cause gut mucosal acidosis at lower bladder pressures, long before the onset of clinical ACS. Uncorrected, it may lead to splanchnic hypoperfusion, ACS, distant organ failure, and death. Prophylactic mesh closure of the abdomen may facilitate the prevention and bedside treatment of IAH and reduce these complications.

Author Commentary by Rao R. Ivatury

In the early 1990s, trauma centers invented "Damage Control Surgery" (DCS).[1] Abbreviated initial laparotomy, resuscitation in ICU, and subsequent return to the operating room for definitive organ repairs to deal with patients presenting in a state of "physiologic exhaustion." DCS, despite benefits, had snares: Unbridled resuscitation fluids, tissue edema and third-space fluid sequestration leading to the syndrome of increased intra-abdominal pressure, or intra-abdominal hypertension. Untreated, the full-blown abdominal compartment syndrome, a morbid multisystem, and multicompartment failure followed. We focused on the interplay of increased intra-abdominal pressure, abdominal compartment syndrome, gut mucosal acidosis, and multiorgan failure and emphasized prophylaxis with open abdomen management (OAM).[2,3] We already had experience with OAM ("laparostomy") having reported on it in approximately 50 patients in 1989 and 1990.

We reported our observations (1992–1997) at the annual assembly of the American Association for the Surgery of Trauma (AAST) in 1997.[4] Our paper advanced two important concepts not emphasized before,[5–7] as Jon Burch mentioned in his discussion: 1. IAH is a pro-drome of ACS. By monitoring bladder pressure (IAP) in these high-risk patients and promptly intervening at the stage of IAH, we may prevent the full syndrome of ACS; splanchnic hypoperfusion and multiorgan failure may commence at much lower IAP than was formerly appreciated. 2. In patients undergoing DCS, "non-closure of the fascia," leaving the abdomen open with a fascial prosthesis may prevent ACS, reduce organ failures, and lead to better survival: one of the first[4,8] to recommend *prophylactic* OAM after DCS. Since then, OAM became an integral part of DCS principles, even though temporary abdominal closure (TAC) varied in its type and form.

Our knowledge of IAH and ACS and the science of OAM continued to be codified by trauma centers. The ensuing results were nothing short of dramatic. Currently, many trauma centers are reporting a vastly reduced prevalence of ACS and improved survival, thanks to these principles. For example, in a prospective, observational study of 478 consecutive patients with OAM for IAH, Cheatham and Safcsak[9] noted that patient survival to hospital discharge increased from 50% to 72% (p = .015). Same-admission primary fascial closure improved from 59% to 81%. A new field of open abdomen and its management was thus born and refined, with improved results.

REFERENCES

1. Schwab CW. Master surgeon lecture: Damage control—20 years of experience. aast.org. Accessed June 2, 2017.
2. Ivatury RR, Simon RJ. Intra-abdominal hypertension. In Ivatury RR, Cayten CG, Eds. *The Textbook of Penetrating Trauma.* Baltimore, MD: Williams & Wilkins, 1996.
3. Ivatury RR, Diebel L, Porter JM, et al. Intra-abdominal hypertension and the abdominal compartment syndrome. *Surg Clin North Am.* 1997; 77(4): 783–800.
4. Ivatury RR, Porter JM, Simon RJ, et al. Intra-abdominal hypertension after life-threatening penetrating abdominal trauma: Prophylaxis, incidence, and clinical relevance to gastric mucosal pH and abdominal compartment syndrome. *J Trauma.* 1998; 44(6): 1016–1021.
5. Burch JM, Ortiz VB, Richardson JR, et al. Abbreviated laparotomy and planned reoperation for critically injured patients. *Ann Surg.* 1992; 215: 476–484.
6. Morris JA Jr., Eddy VA, Blinman TA, et al. The staged celiotomy for trauma: Issues in unpacking and reconstruction. *Ann Surg.* 1993; 217(5): 576–584.
7. Meldrum DR, Moore FA, Moore EE, et al. Prospective characterization and selective management of the abdominal compartment syndrome. *Am J Surg.* 1997; 174(6): 667–672
8. Mayberry JC, Mullins RJ, Crass RA, et al. Prevention of abdominal compartment syndrome by absorbable mesh prosthesis closure. *Arch Surg.* 1997; 132(9): 957–961.
9. Cheatham ML, Safcsak K. Is the evolving management of intra-abdominal hypertension and abdominal compartment syndrome improving survival? *Crit Care Med.* 2010; 38(2): 402–407.

Expert Commentary by Michael L. Cheatham

It can be both fascinating and humbling to study the evolution of surgical management. What we once believed to be *optimal* treatment, is commonly proven to be *suboptimal* in the decades to follow. Few disease processes have evolved at the rate of intra-abdominal hypertension (IAH) and abdominal compartment syndrome (ACS)—clinical entities that were largely unknown until the mid-1990s, yet were widely studied, and their evidence-based management well-defined less than a decade later. Dr. Ivatury and colleagues were present from the beginning of this evolution and accurately predicted 20 years ago the key principles of successful IAH/ACS management that we still rely upon today.

It is important to remember that, while the concept had been envisioned in the 1940s, the term ACS had been described only a few years before this study was published. Many surgeons used the terms ACS, and the much less understood and recognized IAH, interchangeably. Intra-abdominal pressure (IAP) measurements were rarely performed and widely thought unnecessary. Abdominal decompression was considered only if the patient's IAP exceeded 40 mmHg, frequently making it a pre-morbid procedure associated with minimal survival benefit. Some surgeons argued that abdominal decompression should never be performed.

Enter Dr. Ivatury and colleagues, who suggested that IAH was (1) a separate entity from ACS; (2) more common than previously thought; (3) present at lower IAPs than previously described; (4) associated with potentially devastating organ dysfunction; (5) a precursor event to the more detrimental ACS; and (6) treatable through earlier or even prophylactic abdominal decompression. These truths, which we now hold to be standard of care, were both revolutionary and controversial in their time.

While the surgical treatment of IAH/ACS at the time was largely *reactive* (to the presence of organ failure and imminent death), they argued that appropriate management should be *proactive* through preventative serial IAP monitoring and a prophylactic open abdomen in patients at risk. In his response to the discussants, Dr. Ivatury even predicted the now commonplace practice of temporary abdominal closure following damage control laparotomy.

Regrettably, many surgeons to this day fail to heed Dr. Ivatury's recommendation to perform routine IAP measurements, an essential aspect of successful IAH/ACS diagnosis and management. Nevertheless, there is little question that this study, along with a handful of others, has dramatically shaped our current understanding and management of IAH/ACS, stimulating the performance of many subsequent studies that have led to the survival of countless patients who would otherwise have succumbed to this potentially devastating disease process.

Editor Notes: Abdominal hypertension was recognized as a contributor to morbidity and mortality after abdominal catastrophes during the 1990s. This was one of the initial investigations demonstrating the importance of abdominal compartment syndrome as a contributor to physiologic derangements and organ dysfunction after trauma. The benefits of a temporary abdominal closure on the incidence of abdominal hypertension was delineated.

Limitations:

Small population;
Retrospective review of patients who underwent temporary abdominal wall closure or fascial suturing at the discretion of their surgeons;
Lack of blinding;
Huge mortality benefit may have been related to patient selection.

CHAPTER 42

Management of Flail Chest without Mechanical Ventilation

Trinkle JK, Richardson JD, Franz JL, Grover FL, Arom KV,
Holmstrom FM. Ann Thorac Surg 19(4):355–363, 1975

Abstract The pathophysiology of flail chest is usually described only on the basis of paradoxical respiration, ignoring underlying pulmonary contusion. Two groups of comparable patients were treated either with early tracheal intubation and mechanical ventilation (Group 1), or with fluid restriction, diuretics, methylpredinisolone, albumin, vigorous pulmonary toilet, and intercostal nerve blocks, ignoring the paradox and treating only the underlying lung (Group 2). When tracheostomy and mechanical ventilation were not used, the mortality rate went from 21% to 0% (p = 0.01), the complication rate from 100% to 20% (p = 0.005), and the average hospitalization from 31.3 to 9.3 days (p = 0.005). We conclude that most patients with flail chest do not need internal pneumatic stabilization, if the underlying lung is treated appropriately, and that tracheostomy and prolonged mechanical ventilation with a volume respirator, as practiced in most respiratory care centers, is usually a triumph of technique over judgment.

Author Commentary by J. David Richardson

The relevance of this paper may be difficult to comprehend in the second decade of the twenty-first century, but 42 years ago it was revolutionary. To understand its relevance, one needs historical context. Flail chest, prior to about 1950, was treated with various mechanical devices in an attempt to stop paradoxical motion of the chest wall (sandbags taped to the chest, towel clips attached to traction devices, etc.). In 1956, the concept of "internal pneumatic stabilization" was introduced[1] in which patients were sedated, placed on a volume ventilator, kept in a state of respiratory alkalosis with a tracheostomy for periods of weeks to a month, or longer, until the flail healed, and the chest wall stabilized. In 1973, only 2 years before the abovementioned paper was presented, a review stated, "Any treatment short of endotracheal intubation or tracheostomy plus mechanical ventilation almost always proves fatal."[2] The fear was that patients would suddenly decompensate if they were not ventilated.

In San Antonio, prior to this study, patients were managed by a so-called "Respirology Service," and all patients underwent immediate tracheostomy and long-term ventilation. I was a thoracic surgery resident when we excised a sternal chondrosarcoma. The patient was immediately extubated and had a substantial bilateral flail chest but was oxygenating appropriately with adequate pain control. In a contiguous bed was a patient with a small flail segment being ventilated via a tracheostomy tube with nosocomial pneumonia. His diagnosis was made by the Respirology Service by placing two coins (quarters) on each side of his chest and observing whether or not they moved synchronously. When they did not, he had a tracheostomy and ventilator treatment despite normal oxygenation. The results of such treatment regimens were often disastrous: nosocomial pneumonia frequently occurred; barotrauma from the volume ventilation was common with pneumothorax the result. These results often occurred in patients with pre-intubation, normal pulmonary mechanics, and oxygenation.

The San Antonio team had conducted several experimental studies[3-5] on pulmonary contusion, and they suggested underlying lung injury was the real culprit in flail chest. While several of the treatments rendered to our patients were likely unnecessary (methylprednisolone and albumin), good pain control, limited crystalloid resuscitation to avoid worsening the pulmonary contusion, and avoidance of intubation and ventilation proved crucial in obtaining markedly improved results over the previous method of treatment.

The results of this paper changed the management of flail chest almost immediately, and the concept of "internal pneumatic stabilization" faded into oblivion. Interestingly, within the past few years, the dangers of overaggressive flail resuscitation and the pro-inflammatory nature of crystalloid infusion has been "rediscovered."

REFERENCES

1. Avery EE, March ET, Benson DW. Critically crushed chest: A new method of treatment with continuous mechanical hyperventilation to *reduce alkalosis* apnea and internal pneumatic stabilization. *J Thorac Surg.* 1956; 32: 291.
2. Hallstrand HO. Crushing chest injuries. *Int Surg.* 1973; 58: 316.
3. Trinkle JK, Furman RW, Hinshaw MA, et al. Pulmonary contusion: Pathogenesis and effect of various resuscitative measures. *Ann Thorac Surg.* 1973; 16(6): 568.
4. Richardson JD, Franz JL, Grover FL, et al. Pulmonary contusion and hemorrhage: crystalloid versus colloid replacement. *J Surg Res.* 1974; 16: 330.
5. Franz JL, Richardson JD, Grover FL, et al. Effect of methylprednisolone sodium succinate on experimental pulmonary contusion. *J Thorac Cardiovasc Surg.* 1974; 68: 842.

Expert Commentary by Alden H. Harken

If you ask patients (or surgeons) to prioritize the things that they really like to do—breathing is at the top of almost everyone's list. Breathing is relaxing, comfortable, physiologically important, and fun. With almost any other bone, when we break it, we stop using it. You see people walking around all the time with casts on their arms. They are comfortable because they are not using their broken arms.

With a rib, it is not so easy. For a surgeon, it is gratifying to control pain. It requires a big hit to break several ribs—and it hurts—a lot. So, traditionally we anesthetized the patient and told the patient's family (and ourselves) that we were "internally splinting the chest."

Safe anesthesia obligated tracheal intubation with its attendant continuous aspiration and compromised pulmonary toilet. Liberal fluid resuscitation was the hallmark of a first-class trauma program. When this aggressive fluid therapy exacerbated the local edema in the underlying traumatized lung, we signed this out as "patient disease" at our Morbidity and Mortality conferences. And, when the continuous aspiration seeded the fluid-flooded zone of contused lung, provoking pneumonia, we complained to the respiratory therapists about suboptimal care.

Then 45 years ago, along came Trinkle and his Texas cowboy colleagues, who specifically identified each of these glaringly apparent therapeutic insults and decided to buck tradition. They compared their past experience of anesthetizing and intubating patients with "flail chests" to a new group in which they restricted fluid, avoided intubation and tracheostomy, and controlled pain with individual intercostal nerve blocks.

When tracheostomy and mechanical ventilation were not used, the mortality rate went from 21% to 0% ($p = 0.01$), the complication rate from 100% to 20% ($p = 0.005$), and the average hospitalization from 31.3 to 9.3 days. With results like these, we don't need statistics—and a prospective, randomized trial would be unethical.

One just wonders how many other glaringly obvious ill-advised traditions we are still inflicting upon our unsuspecting and trusting patients.

Editor Notes: Prior to this study, internal pneumatic stabilization (tracheostomy, mechanical ventilation) was the standard management of flail chest. After this report revealed a lower mortality (21%–0%) and morbidity with this management protocol, the policy of pulmonary toilet and pain control with selective use of mechanical ventilation became the standard of care following severe chest trauma.

Limitations:

Historical control group;
Small population size.

CHAPTER 43

Rib Fractures in the Elderly

Bulger EM, Arneson MA, Mock CN, Jurkovich GJ.
J Trauma 48(6):1040–1046; discussion 1046–1047, 2000

Abstract   In this study, we sought to define the problem by exploring the impact of age on outcome after rib fractures, defining the relationship between number of rib fractures and outcome, and evaluating the influence of analgesic technique on outcome. This was a retrospective chart review over 10 years from Harborview Medical Center. The results demonstrated significantly worse outcome for patients over age 65 and raised awareness that even a limited number of rib fractures was associated with an increased risk of pneumonia in this patient population. The limitations of retrospective data did not allow us to draw conclusions about the influence of analgesia approach, and we suggested in the discussion that further prospective analysis was needed. This led us to conduct a subsequent randomized controlled trial of epidural analgesia versus intravenous narcotics, which demonstrated that the epidural approach was associated with a twofold reduction in the risk of pneumonia and 2 fewer days on the ventilator for ventilated patients.[1] We also explored the contraindications to epidural use in trauma patients.[2]

Background   We sought to ascertain the extent to which advanced age influences the morbidity and mortality after rib fractures (fxs), to define the relationship between number of rib fractures and morbidity and mortality, and to evaluate the influence of analgesic technique on outcome.

Methods   A retrospective cohort study involving all 277 patients ≥ 65 years old with rib fxs admitted to a level I trauma center over 10 years was undertaken. The control group consisted of 187 randomly selected patients, 18–64 years old, with rib fxs admitted over the same time period. Outcomes included pulmonary complications, number of ventilator days, length of intensive care unit and hospital stay (LOS), disposition, and mortality. The specific analgesic technique used was also examined.

Results   The two groups had similar mean number of rib fxs (3.6 elderly vs. 4.0 young), mean chest Abbreviated Injury Scores (3.0 vs. 3.0), and mean Injury Severity Score (20.7 vs. 21.4). However, mean number of ventilator days (4.3 vs. 3.1), intensive care unit days (6.1 vs. 4.0), and LOS (15.4 vs. 10.7 days) were longer for the elderly patients. Pneumonia occurred in 31% of elderly versus 17% of young (p < 0.01), and mortality was 22% for the elderly versus 10% for the young (p < 0.01). Mortality and pneumonia rates increased as the number of rib fxs increased with and odds ratio for death of 1.19 and for pneumonia of 1.16 per each additional rib fracture (p < 0.001). The use of epidural analgesia in the elderly (LOS >2 days) was associated with a 10% mortality versus 16% without the use of an epidural (p = 0.28). In the younger group (LOS >2 days), mortality with and without the use of an epidural was 0% and 5%, respectively.

Conclusions   Elderly patients who sustain blunt chest trauma with rib fxs have twice the mortality and thoracic morbidity of younger patients with similar injuries. For each additional rib fracture in the elderly, mortality increases by 19% and the risk of pneumonia by 27%. As the number of rib fractures increases, there is a significant increase in morbidity and mortality in both groups, but with different patterns for each group. Further prospective study is needed to determine the utility of epidural analgesia in this population.

Author Commentary by Eileen M. Bulger

This paper was inspired by a patient who I cared for as a surgery resident and died as a result of his rib fractures. The patient was an elderly gentleman who was living independently and fell from a ladder at his home. He suffered four rib fractures on the right side with a pneumothorax, which required a chest tube. He had no major medical comorbidities and was admitted to a thoracic surgeon in a non-trauma center. He was treated with IV narcotics for management of his pain. Over the next few days, he became increasingly delirious and subsequently had an aspiration event requiring intubation and transfer to the ICU. He then developed a nosocomial pneumonia, which progressed to septic shock resulting in his death. I was struck by the fact that this isolated injury had led to such a devastating outcome.

Over the last 17 years, our group has continued to explore the process of care to improve outcomes for all patients admitted with rib fractures and recently published a review of our comprehensive inpatient rib fracture protocol, which was developed as a quality improvement project at Harborview.[3] As the geriatric population in the United States continues to increase, our trauma centers are faced with the challenges of a growing number of elderly patients admitted with what may seem like minor injuries, but have a very poor outcome. It is our hope that this work will lead to increased awareness of the importance of a standardized, multidisciplinary approach to these patients to optimize outcomes.

REFERENCES

1. Bulger EM, Edwards T, Klotz P, Jurkovich GJ. Epidural analgesia improves outcome after multiple rib fractures. *Surgery*. 2004; 136(2): 426–430.
2. Bulger EM, Edwards WT, de Pinto M, Klotz P, Jurkovich GJ. Indications and contraindications for thoracic epidural analgesia in multiply injured patients. *Acute Pain*. 2008; 10(1): 15–22.
3. Witt CE, Bulger EM. Comprehensive approach to the management of the patient with multiple rib fractures: A review and introduction of a bundled rib fracture management protocol. *Trauma Surg Acute Care Open*. 2017; 2(1): e000064. (tsaco.bmj.com)

Expert Commentary by J. Wayne Meredith

The paper "Rib Fractures in the Elderly" is an important paper in our understanding of blunt trauma, especially blunt trauma in the elderly. Even today, looking back to the end of the twentieth century when these data were collected, it is easy to appreciate how this paper quantified the magnitude of the impact of rib fractures and the extent of the impact of multiple rib fractures on the mortality and morbidity of blunt trauma patients. Looking back on those almost 20 years, it is helpful to place this article in the context of the time in which it was published. At the end of the twentieth century, trauma centers were well-established across the country but mostly in places that had historically performed predominantly penetrating trauma, and the prevalence of large trauma centers performing and studying blunt trauma was much lower than today. The interest in and the prevalence of geriatric patients was reaching the early phase of the baby boom expansion. At that time, many trauma surgeons equated severity of injury, intentionally or unintentionally or subconsciously, with energy absorption alone. A single or a few multiple rib fractures, especially in an elderly patient whose ribs are brittle, was not considered always a sign of an absorption of a great deal of energy and, therefore, subconsciously not severe. However, the impact in these elderly patients of multiple rib fractures on their physiology and their ability to maintain pulmonary secretions, and so on, was profound and underappreciated until this article.

This article first set forth a new perception of the reality that rib fractures in elderly patients, though an injury that required little energy to create, was a sign of a more physiologically impactful injury, than a similar set of rib fractures in a young patient, that is roughly linearly associated with the number of fractures. It did not require lung contusion for this impact to be realized.

These observations have had a profound impact on our understanding on the level of care needed for elderly patients, both in terms of what level of trauma center in which they should be treated as well as within that trauma center where they should receive their care. In addition, this is one of a few papers that drew attention to the importance of appropriate pain management in patients with rib fractures, which has been an additional significant contribution of this paper. However, I would say its seminal contribution is the realization of the importance of the number of rib fractures and morbidity to trauma patients and its importance in the geriatric population.

Editor Notes: This paper retrospectively reviewed the outcomes of patients with rib fractures and found a much higher morbidity and mortality in individuals over 64 years old, when compared to younger trauma victims. A very important finding was that each additional rib fracture was associated with a nearly 20% increase in mortality, as well a significant increase in the incidence of pneumonia and ARDS. This study led to our current more intensive approach to management of chest wall injury in older patients.

Limitations:

Retrospective analysis;
Single center experience over a prolonged time period (10 years);
Limited population size;
Cohort study so comparison group was matched, and 65 years was an arbitrary
    threshold for analysis.

CHAPTER 44

Efficacy of Short-Course Antibiotic Prophylaxis after Penetrating Intestinal Injury: A Prospective Randomized Trial

Dellinger EP, Wertz MJ, Lennard ES, Oreskovich MR. Arch Surg 121(1):23–30, 1986

Abstract   Infection is the leading cause of morbidity and mortality occurring more than 48 hours after penetrating abdominal injury. Antibiotics are routinely administered to patients with penetrating intestinal injuries and are usually given for 5 days or more. We randomized 116 patients with confirmed penetrating injuries of the colon and/or small bowel to receive either 12 hours or 5 days of antibiotics. Age, sex, weapon, severity of injury, and other risk factors were evenly distributed between groups. Twenty-one patients (18%) developed trauma-related infections, 28 (24%) any infection, and three (2.6%) died. There were no significant differences between groups in any category of outcome. For patients with penetrating intestinal or colonic injury, a 12-hour course of antibiotics is as effective as a 5-day course and has the advantage of lower cost and, theoretically, fewer side effects.

Author Commentary by E. Patchen Dellinger

Surgical site infection (SSI) has been a concern of surgeons since the earliest days of the profession. Handwashing and antisepsis were first introduced in the 1800s and surgical gloves in the 1920s. Antibiotics became available in the mid-twentieth century, and animal experiments by Miles,[1] Burke,[2] Alexander,[3] and Edlich[4] between 1957 and 1973 showed that administration of antibiotics prior to incision could prevent many SSIs. The trials by Bernard[5] in 1964 and Polk[6] in 1969 showed that this applied to humans as well for scheduled cases. Most early trials gave a dose of antibiotic before incision and two more over the next 12 hours. However, as early as 1976, trials demonstrating the efficacy of single doses had been published, and multiple trials between 1972 and 1986 demonstrated equal efficacy for shorter courses of antibiotic compared to longer ones.[7–12] Despite this, the tendency of surgeons to prolong "prophylactic" antibiotic administration for many days has persisted, and a study in 2005 showed that 50% of patients in the United States were getting more than 36 hours of "prophylactic" antibiotic.[13] In the meantime, in the 1970s, as the principles of effective care of trauma patients were being developed, it was assumed that we could not give "prophylactic" antibiotics to trauma patients, especially those with penetrating injuries, because the injury occurred before antibiotics could be given, and thus we were "treating" infection rather than preventing it. Nevertheless, a retrospective review by Fullen[14] in 1972 showed that the timing of antibiotic administration did make a difference in penetrating abdominal trauma patients, and earlier administration was more effective than later administration. Indeed, while antibiotics cannot be given before the injury, they can be given before the incision and provide protection for the exposed abdominal wall tissues in that incision. The assumption continued to be that, because they were given after the injury, the duration needed to be prolonged. In this setting, our group at Harborview Medical Center carried out the prospective trial described above comparing 12 hours to 5 days of antibiotics for patients with documented intestinal injuries and demonstrated that there was no benefit to the prolonged duration.[15] These results were later confirmed at New York Hospital.[16] Subsequently, we also conducted a multicenter trial of duration of prophylactic antibiotics for open fractures and showed that there was no benefit to 5 days compared with a single dose of a long-acting cephalosporin (effectively 12–18 hours).[17] The tendency for physicians to prolong the duration of antibiotic administration continues in the absence of its value in many circumstances. Subsequent studies have shown that shorter durations are appropriate for pneumonia[18] and intra-abdominal infection.[19] Antibiotics get continued for fever but they are not antipyretics. Antibiotics get continued to make physicians, patients, and families feel better as tranquilizers. But this continued, ineffective use increases the risk of adverse reactions, development of resistance and superinfection, and *C. difficile* colitis. Antibiotic administration should be kept as short as possible for our patients based on data such as those cited above.

REFERENCES

1. Miles A, Miles E, Burke J. The value and duration of defence reactions of the skin to the primary lodgement of bacteria. *Br J Exp Pathol.* 1957; 38: 79–96.
2. Burke JF. The effective period of preventive antibiotic action in experimental incisions and dermal lesions. *Surgery.* 1961; 50: 161–168.
3. Alexander J, Altemeier W. Penicillin prophylaxis of experimental staphylococcal wound infections. *Surg Gyn Ob.* 1965; 120: 243–255.
4. Edlich R, Smith Q, Edgerton M. Resistance of the surgical wound to antimicrobial prophylaxis and its mechanisms of development. *Am J Surg.* 1973; 126: 583–591.
5. Bernard H, Cole W. The prophylaxis of surgical infection: The effect of prophylactic antimicrobial drugs on the incidence of infection following potentially contaminated operations. *Surgery.* 1964; 56: 151–157.
6. Polk HC, Jr, Lopez-Mayor JF. Postoperative wound infection: A prospective study of determinant factors and prevention. *Surgery.* 1969; 66: 97–103.
7. Strachan CJ, Black J, Powis SJ, et al. Prophylactic use of cephazolin against wound sepsis after cholecystectomy. *Br Med J.* 1977; 1: 1254–1256.
8. Pollard JP, Hughes SP, Scott JE, Evans MJ, Benson MK. Antibiotic prophylaxis in total hip replacement. *Br Med J.* 1979; 1: 707–709.

9. Mendelson J, Portnoy J, De Saint Victor JR, Gelfand MM. Effect of single and multidose cephradine prophylaxis on infectious morbidity of vaginal hysterectomy. *Obstet Gynecol.* 1979; 53: 31–35.

10. Goldmann DA, Hopkins CC, Karchmer AW, et al. Cephalothin prophylaxis in cardiac valve surgery: A prospective, double-blind comparison of two-day and six-day regimens. *J Thorac Cardiovasc Surg.* 1977; 73: 470–479.

11. DiPiro J, Cheung R, Bowden T, Jr. Single dose systemic antibiotic prophylaxis of surgical wound infections. *Am J Surg.* 1986; 152: 552–559.

12. Conte JE, Jr., Cohen SN, Roe BB, Elashoff RM. Antibiotic prophylaxis and cardiac surgery: A prospective double-blind comparison of single-dose versus multiple-dose regimens. *Ann Intern Med.* 1972; 76: 943–949.

13. Bratzler DW, Houck PM, Richards C, et al. Use of antimicrobial prophylaxis for major surgery: Baseline results from the national surgical infection prevention project. *Arch Surg.* 2005; 140: 174–182.

14. Fullen WD, Hunt J, Altemeier WA. Prophylactic antibiotics in penetrating wounds of the abdomen. *J Trauma.*1972; 12: 282–289.

15. Dellinger EP, Wertz MJ, Lennard ES, Oreskovich MR. Efficacy of short-course antibiotic prophylaxis after penetrating intestinal injury: A prospective randomized trial. *Arch Surg.* 1986; 121: 23–30.

16. Bozorgzadeh A, Pizzi WF, Barie PS, et al. The duration of antibiotic administration in penetrating abdominal trauma. *Am J Surg.* 1999; 177: 125–131.

17. Dellinger EP, Caplan ES, Weaver LD, et al. Duration of preventive antibiotic administration for open extremity fractures. *Arch Surg.* 1988; 123: 333–339.

18. Chastre J, Wolff M, Fagon JY, et al. Comparison of 8 vs 15 days of antibiotic therapy for ventilator-associated pneumonia in adults: a randomized trial. *JAMA.* 2003; 290:2588–2598.

19. Sawyer RG, Claridge JA, Nathens AB, et al. Trial of short-course antimicrobial therapy for intraabdominal infection. *N Engl J Med.* 2015; 372: 1996–2005. doi:10.1056/NEJMoa1411162.

Expert Commentary by Philip S. Barie

In the early 1980s, penetrating abdominal trauma (PAT) was more prevalent than now, and major trauma centers were awash. Infection was recognized as dangerous, but the role of anaerobes in establishing mixed infection and intraperitoneal abscess formation had been observed experimentally only recently[1] and had not been translated widely into clinical practice. Indeed, this writer recalls that, when as a junior resident in 1977–1978, the empiric regimen for sepsis on the surgical service was a combination of cephalothin and gentamicin, which conferred no activity against gut-derived anaerobes. Anti-anaerobic agents were available (e.g., chloramphenicol, clindamycin, various tetracyclines), but not used routinely.

Bartlett and Onderdonk, working with Gorbach in his Tufts laboratory, established a reproducible rat bacterial peritonitis model, demonstrating that aerobes and anaerobes act synergistically to cause abscess, and that coverage against both was optimal.[2] Although Miles and Burke had defined a 3- to 4-hour period following bacterial inoculation of skin/soft tissue, during which a single dose of antibiotic was effective,[3,4] it was commonplace to treat therapeutically with antibiotics for days (4–12 days in contemporary publications).[5]

In preliminary work published in 1982,[5] Oreskovich et al. randomized 82 patients with PAT to receive either a single dose of doxycycline and 12 hours of penicillin (PCN) G or those two agents for a total of 5 days; 47 patients had a hollow viscus injury. There were 7 infections noted overall in the hollow viscus subset (4 in the 12-hour group), so there was no signal of lack of efficacy of the short-course group, although the study was underpowered.

In the seminal work feted herein,[6] 116 patients (also underpowered) were randomized either to the same regimen as previously, or later in the study, high-dose cefoxitin monotherapy for either 12 hours or 5 days), now with a placebo control for additional doses in the 12-hour group. Cefoxitin (introduced in the United States in 1980) certainly was an advance as was the placebo control, but infection rates hovered around 25% overall. A sample size of about 660 subjects would be required to detect a 25% reduction of infection risk with 80% power and 95% confidence. Changing the agent mid-study was highly problematic, reducing power further. Was this study the state of the art in 1986? Your writer would argue perhaps not, but it was first to support short-duration prophylaxis.

In 1984, Nichols et al. published[7] a paper that also merits attention. The study included 619 patients who were enrolled to receive cefoxitin plus placebo or gentamicin plus clindamycin for 5 days. Of these patients, 145 patients randomized intraoperatively (after hollow viscus injury was identified), thereby enriching the population under study, for the condition under study, through the use (novel at the time) of a handheld calculator for allocation. Nichols et al. found the infection rates to be 20%–23% (p = NS), but contributed greatly to understanding the risks through the (unusual for the time) use of multivariable analysis. Nichols et al. were first to show that risk for infection after PAT increased with the number of organs injured, with the number of units of blood/blood products transfused, creation of an ostomy, and increasing age. Notably colon injury per se was not an identified risk factor, a (correct) finding that was surprising at the time.

Taken together, and with the 20 or so similar studies that would be published in the ensuing two decades, what was "learned?" Patients with PAT, but no hollow viscus injury, need a single dose of preoperative antibiotic prophylaxis. Period. Provided operation occurs within 12 hours (the current defined interval after which colonization is presumed to become invasive infection), patients with a hollow viscus injury need only 24 hours of prophylaxis *even if there is a colon injury.* Pre- or intraoperative shock is irrelevant, except in the case of massive ongoing blood loss, during which intraoperative re-dosing should occur based on the pharmacokinetics of the agent administered. Why do I say learned, parenthetically? It seems that every succeeding generation of surgeons forgets these lessons. In my travels, any number of excuses come up to prolong antibiotic prophylaxis (and not just for PAT). Colon injury, shock, volume of blood loss, volume of enteric contents in the peritoneal cavity ... all are put forth. None of them matter.

REFERENCES

1. Altemeier WA. Sepsis in surgery: Presidential address. *Arch Surg*.1982; 117: 107–112.
2. Bartlett JG, Onderdonk AB, Louie T, et al. A review: Lessons from an animal model of intra-abdominal sepsis. *Arch Surg*. 1978; 113: 853–857.
3. Miles AA, Miles EM, Burke J. The value and duration of defense reactions of the skin to the primary lodgment of bacteria. *Br J Exp Pathol*. 1957; 38: 79–96.
4. Burke JF. The effective period of preventive antibiotic action in experimental incisions and dermal lesions. *Surgery*. 1961; 50: 161–168.
5. Oreskovich MR, Dellinger EP, Lennard ES, et al. Duration of preventive antibiotic administration for penetrating abdominal trauma. *Arch Surg*. 1982; 117: 200–205.
6. Dellinger EP, Wertz MJ, Lennard ES, Oreskovich MR. Efficacy of short-course antibiotic prophylaxis after penetrating intestinal injury. *Arch Surg*. 1986; 121; 23–30.
7. Nichols RL, Smith JW, Klein DB, et al. Risk of infection after penetrating abdominal trauma. *N Engl J Med*. 1984; 311: 1065–1070.

Editor Notes: Prior to this investigation it was routine for patients to receive a prolonged "prophylactic" antibiotic course for many days after penetrating abdominal injuries. This randomized trial of patients with intestinal trauma revealed no difference in infectious outcomes, related to the length of postoperative antibiotics (12 hours versus 5 days).

Limitations:

Not double-blinded study;
Relatively small population (n = 116) underpowered to prove equivalency;
Variable antibiotic coverage;
No long-term follow-up in 11%.

CHAPTER 45

A Multicenter, Randomized, Controlled Clinical Trial of Transfusion Requirements in Critical Care. Transfusion Requirements in Critical Care Investigators, Canadian Critical Care Trials Group

Hébert PC, Wells G, Blajchman MA, Marshall J, Martin C, Pagliarello G, Tweeddale M, Schweitzer I, Yetisir E. N Engl J Med 340(6):409–417, 1999

Abstract   It has been 18 years since the publication of the Transfusion Requirements in Critical Care (TRICC) trial.[1] Since then, 20 randomized trials of transfusion triggers have been published since, all generally demonstrating that a restrictive transfusion strategy decreases red cell transfusions by 50% without any negative consequences on clinically important outcomes.[2] If anything, outcomes were better in some subgroups in the restrictive arm.

Background   To determine whether a restrictive strategy of red cell transfusion and a liberal strategy produced equivalent results in critically ill patients, we compared the rates of death from all causes at 30 days and the severity of organ dysfunction.

Methods   We enrolled 838 critically ill patients with euvolemia after initial treatment who had hemoglobin concentrations of less than 9.0 g per deciliter within 72 hours after admission to the intensive care unit. Of the total, we randomly assigned 418 patients to a restrictive strategy of transfusion, in which red cells were transfused if the hemoglobin concentration dropped below 7.0 g per deciliter and hemoglobin concentrations were maintained at 7.0 g–9.0 g per deciliter and 420 patients to a liberal strategy, in which transfusions were given when the hemoglobin concentration fell below 10.0 g per deciliter and hemoglobin concentrations were maintained at 10.0 g–12.0 g per deciliter.

Results   Overall, 30-day mortality was similar in the two groups (18.7% vs. 23.3%, p = 0.11). However, the rates were significantly lower with the restrictive transfusion strategy among patients who were less acutely ill—those with an Acute Physiology and Chronic Health Evaluation II score of ≤ 20 (8.7% in the restrictive-strategy group and 16.1% in the liberal strategy group; p = 0.03)—and among patients who were less than 55 years of age (5.7% and 13.0%, respectively; p = 0.02), but not among patients with clinically significant cardiac disease (20.5%

and 22.9%, respectively; $p = 0.69$). The mortality rate during hospitalization was significantly lower in the restrictive-strategy group (22.3% vs. 28.1%, $p = 0.05$).

Conclusions   A restrictive strategy of red cell transfusion is at least as effective as, and possibly superior to, a liberal transfusion strategy in critically ill patients, with the possible exception of patients with acute myocardial infarction and unstable angina.

Author Commentary by Paul C. Hébert

The journey started in 1991, where as a research fellow, I wondered about exploring whether a much more liberal strategy (threshold held greater than 12.0 g/dL versus a much more restrictive one [transfusion threshold less than 7.0 g/dL]) would improve oxygen delivery sufficiently to save lives of supply dependent patients with septic shock. I wrote the study as part of a clinical trials course for my master's degree. I continued to refine the protocol over the next 2 years. Then, I presented the study at the Canadian Critical Care Trials Groups (CCCTG) in the spring of 1993.

During my presentation to Canada's leading intensivists, I quickly found that every part of the trial would be scrutinized and questioned. My colleagues were far less interested in the concept of driving up oxygen delivery to save lives but far more interested in simply understanding how and when to transfuse red cells. They then pointed out that red cell transfusions had important effects on immune response and predisposed to infections and may well increase the rates of acute lung injury. Through our discussions, it became clear that both arms of the trial had its proponents. Unfortunately, it also became clear that each side was entrenched in their respective views and practices. The discussion became very animated with one side stating the other was engaged in malpractice. Then, one wise member of our group stood up to say that the divergent views in a largely data free zone were in fact exactly why we needed to do the trial. And thereafter, we had a few more hours of constructive debate, and with each intervention, the trial was made better.

After assembling a team of critical care physicians, a world class biostatistician, Dr. George Wells, and a transfusion medicine expert, Morris Blajchman, we received a Medical Research Council grant on our first submission. And then, we implemented the project, attempting to recruit 2,300 patients over the next 5 years. After 4 years, fewer patients and physicians were agreeing to participate in the study. Canadians were hearing about contaminated blood scandals on a daily basis because of an ongoing Royal Commission (equivalent to Senate hearings or investigations in the United States). Despite our best efforts, we were unable to increase enrollment rates. We finally decided to close out the study after 838 patients, an insufficient number to properly ensure that both arms of the trial were equivalent.

Several months later, the trial statistician and I proceeded to go through the primary analysis together, and to our surprise, the restrictive group seemed to do a bit better. I could not believe my eyes. I asked to check the coding. Could we have mislabeled the group? He said no. He had already checked. And then, I wanted to know a lot more. Were there subgroups more affected than others? Were the results consistent? What about secondary outcomes? What about high-risk groups, like patients with heart disease? The enthusiasm of that day is still with me. To be looking at data that no one else has seen! And especially, with results that were so unexpected. We thought we were going to find nothing in an underpowered study. Instead, we were looking at data from a groundbreaking study.

Almost 10 years after the first protocol draft, several hundred of us completed groundbreaking work. It then took over another decade and many other studies with similar findings before red cell transfusion practice changed. It is personally very gratifying to have been part of such an important team effort, especially as a young scientist. I only hope our next generation considers a career in clinical research.

LESSONS

1. Great scientific work is best done collectively within research networks.
2. Being open to feedback and ideas is an essential skill set for modern scientists.
3. Persevere, don't get too close to your hypothesis, and let the data speak for itself.
4. Mentorship is a key ingredient to success.

REFERENCES

1. Hébert PC, Wells G, Blajchman MA, et al. For the Canadian critical care trials group. *Transfusion Requirements in Critical Care: A Multicentre Randomized Controlled Clinical Trial. N Engl J Med.* 1999; 340: 409–417.
2. Carson JL, Stanworth SJ, Roubinian N, et al. Clinical trials evaluating red blood cell Transfusion thresholds: An updated systematic review and subgroups including cardiovascular disease cochrane database. *Syst Rev.* 2016; 10: CD002042. Review (update forthcoming).

Expert Commentary by Martin A. Schreiber

The study by Hébert et al., commonly known as the TRICC trial, has been one of the most influential papers written during our lifetime. This study resulted in a substantial reduction in red blood cell (RBC) transfusions throughout the world potentially even threatening the viability of blood banks.

The study was a prospective, randomized, multicenter trial performed in 25 ICUs in Canada between the years 1994 and 1997. Patients randomized to a restrictive strategy had a transfusion threshold of 7.0 g/dL and a goal hemoglobin between 7.0 and 9.0 g/dL versus a liberal strategy with a transfusion threshold of 10.0 g/dL and a goal hemoglobin between 10 and 12 g/dL.

Patients randomized to the restrictive strategy received less than half the number of blood transfusions, and 33% avoided any RBC transfusion at all. All of the patients in the liberal group were transfused at least 1 unit of RBCs. The randomization was continued while patients were in the ICU only.

Patients who were randomized to the restrictive group had a lower mortality at hospital discharge. However, mortality was not significantly different at the predefined primary outcome period of 30 days. The subgroups of patients with APACHE II scores ≤ 20 and age < 55 years did have lower mortality at 30 days. Cardiac events, including pulmonary edema and myocardial infarction were more common in the liberal group during the ICU stay. There was no difference in outcomes among the patients with underlying cardiac disease.

While interpreting the results of this study, there are several important factors to consider. The initial power analysis was for 1,620 patients; however, the study was stopped after 838 patients due to low enrollment indicating that it was likely underpowered, and the potential exists that there could have been a difference in the primary outcome if the study went to completion. Also, the RBCs utilized in the study were not leukodepleted raising the possibility that it is not widely applicable. The study only included normovolemic patients who weren't bleeding. Finally, the authors did not provide data on the age of blood, which could play a role in the negative outcomes seen in the liberal group.

Despite the limitations of the study, it served to eliminate many fallacies related to transfusion medicine. Previous to the TRICC trial, many practitioners transfused to a goal hemoglobin of 10 g/dL based on minimal data. This practice was especially pronounced in patients with underlying cardiac disease in whom a hemoglobin of 10 g/dL was almost mandatory. This study revealed no benefit to these practices and even suggested that they may be detrimental and certainly unnecessarily waste a very precious resource.

Editor Notes: This classic paper altered our approach to transfusion in the critically ill adult population. In a meticulously performed multicenter randomized trial of 838 patients, a restrictive (Hb 7–9 g/dL) transfusion strategy was shown to lower mortality, when compared to a liberal (Hb 10–12 g/dL) transfusion strategy (22% vs. 28%, p = 0.05).

Limitations:

Patients with acute cardiac ischemic events and acute GI bleeds were excluded; Adult population only.

CHAPTER 46

Early Predictors of Postinjury Multiple Organ Failure

Sauaia A, Moore FA, Moore EE, Haenel JB, Read RA,
Lezotte DC. Arch Surg 129(1):39–45, 1994

Abstract   In the late 1980s, the Denver Multiple Organ Failure (MOF) database
was developed to prospectively characterize postinjury MOF. At this time, MOF
was a frequent, poorly understood and highly morbid syndrome. This manuscript
was the first database analysis and set the stage for the authors' future MOF research
efforts.[1] It showed that MOF could be accurately predicted within 12 hours based
on age, injury severity, early blood transfusion requirements, and shock severity.

Objective   To find a predictive model for postinjury multiple organ failure.

Design   A 3-year cohort study ending December 1992 (first year:
retrospective; last 2 years: prospective).

Setting   Denver General Hospital (CO) is a regional level I trauma center.

Patients   Consecutive trauma patients with an Injury Severity Score (ISS)
greater than 15, with an age greater than 16 years, and who survived longer than
24 hours. Stepwise logistic regression analysis was performed in all patients
($n = 394$), in the subgroup of patients with 0–12 hours, plus 12–24 hours base
deficit (BD) results ($n = 220$), and in a second subgroup of patients with
BD plus lactate results at 0–12 hours and 12–24 hours ($n = 106$).

Main Outcome   Postinjury MOF.

Results   The following variables were identified as independent predictors of MOF
in the analysis of all patients: age more than 55 years, ISS greater than or equal to 25,
and more than 6 units (U) of red blood cells in the first 12 hours after admission
(U RBC/12 hours). In the subgroup with BD results, the same analysis identified age
greater than 55 years, greater than 6 U RBC/12 hours, and BD greater than 8 mEq/L
(0–12 hours), while in the last subgroup analysis including BD and lactate results,
greater than 6 U RBC/12 hours, BD greater than 8 mEq/L (0–12 hours), and lactate
greater than 2.5 mmol/L (12–24 hours) were independently associated with MOF.

Conclusions   Age greater than 55 years, ISS greater than or equal to 25, and greater than 6 U RBC/12 hours are early independent predictors of MOF. Subgroup analyses indicate that BD and lactate levels may add substantial predictive value. Moreover, these results emphasize the predominant role of the initial insult in the pathogenesis of postinjury MOF.

Author Commentary by Frederick A. Moore

The data emphasized the importance of the initial insult and identified the shock to be a potential modifiable risk factor. As a result, a resuscitation proto- col was implemented, refined, and studied. This led to a robust characterization of the emerging epidemic of the abdominal compartment syndrome followed by fundamental changes in initial care of severely bleeding patients that have largely eliminated this iatrogenic MOF phenotype.[2] Additionally, MOF was identified to be a bimodal phenomenon with early and late MOF having differ- ent predictors.[3]

Based on these and other contemporary data, a new MOF paradigm of dysregu- lated immunity was proposed and conceptualized to be a systemic inflamma- tory response syndrome (SIRS) followed by a compensatory anti-inflammatory response syndrome (CARS). After successful resuscitation, patients develop SIRS (predominantly an innate immune response). Endogenous damage- associated molecular patterns (DAMPs—e.g., HMGB), or exogenous pathogen- associated molecular patterns (PAMPs—e.g., endotoxin), signaling through pattern recognition receptors (e.g., toll-like receptors) activate inflammation signaling via pro-inflammatory transcription factors (e.g., NF-kB) that activate overlapping cascades of other inflammatory mediators, effector cells and, at the same time, activate endothelial cell dysfunction and prothrombotic events. If severe, the end-result is fulminant early MOF. Based on simultaneous studies of neutrophils (PMNs), the "two-hit" hypothesis was proposed and subsequently validated.

This led to in-depth explorations of classic, G protein-coupled receptor mecha- nisms of PMN priming and activation. Fortunately, most patients with SIRS survive to progress into delayed CARS (principally a depressed adaptive immune response). This was characterized to include increased lymphocyte and dendritic cell apoptosis, macrophage paralysis, increased regulatory T cells, decreased antigen presentation, suppressed T cell proliferation, and a shift from type 1 helper T cell (TH1) to TH2 lymphocyte phenotype. If severe, CARS pro- motes nosocomial infections, which cause late sepsis-induced MOF.

Finally, the observation early blood transfusions were a consistent, indepen- dent, and strong predictor for early MOF focused research on determining the harmful effects of blood transfusions.[4] While other investigators studied the immunosuppressive of blood and its role in causing nosocomial infections, the Denver investigators uniquely identified that "old blood" amplified SIRS and that with blood storage, cell wall degradation produced pro-inflammatory lipids (e.g., platelet activating factor) that serve as PMN priming agents in early MOF pathogenesis. The Denver MOF database has continued to accrue data through today and the dataset has been incorporated into other MOF databases. The ongoing prospective characterization of the evolving epidemiology of MOF has led to numerous novel observations that have directed several team science efforts the elucidating the complex mechanisms involved in the pathophysiology of MOF.[5]

REFERENCES

1. Moore FA, Moore EE. Evolving concepts in the pathogenesis of post injury multiple organ failure. *Surg Clin North Am.* 1995; 75: 257–277.
2. Balogh Z, McKinley BA, Cox CS, Allen SJ, Cocanour CS, Kozar RA, Moore EE, Miller CC, Weisbrodt NW, Moore FA. Abdominal compartment syndrome: The cause or effect of postinjury multiple organ failure. *Shock.* 2003; 20(6): 483–492.
3. Moore FA, Sauaia A, Moore EE, Haenel JB, Burch JM, Lezotte DC. Postinjury multiple organ failure: A bimodal phenomenon. *J Trauma.* 1996; 40(4): 501–512.
4. Moore FA, Moore EE, Sauaia A. Blood transfusion: An independent risk factor for postinjury multiple organ failure. *Arch Surg.* 1997; 132(6): 620–625.
5. Moore FA, Moore EE, Billiar TR, Vodovotz V, Anirban Banerjee A, Moldawer LL. The role of NIGMS P50 sponsored team science in our understanding of multiple organ failure. *J Trauma Acute Care Surg.* 2017; 83(3): 520–531.

Expert Commentary by Addison K. May

What seems clear and logical looking retrospectively, is rarely so when looking prospectively. This certainly holds true when considering our understanding of post-traumatic multiple organ failure. The landmark 1994 publication by Sauaia and colleagues helped to shift the paradigm from occult infection to tissue injury, shock, and hypoperfusion as the etiologic insults causing post-traumatic MOF.[1] For those who trained after the 1990s, a little historical context is required to understand the importance of this shift.

When this study was published, the Apple Macintosh personal computer had been available for 10 years, introduced in 1984. The Internet was not widely used until the following year, 1995. The American College of Surgeons Committee on Trauma verification/consultation system for hospitals had been introduced just 7 years earlier.[2] The American Board of Surgery had formally recognized Surgical Critical Care as a subspecialty in 1986, but the period during which surgeons could grandfather into it was only just ending.[3] TNF and IL-6 had been clearly characterized for less than 10 years.[4,5] Abdominal compartment syndrome as an entity in trauma resuscitation and the "damage control" approach to manage exsanguination in penetrating abdominal trauma had been just described.[6,7]

While CT imaging was readily available, it was slow enough that the decision on when to perform a diagnostic peritoneal lavage (DPL), in lieu of a CT, was often quite difficult. Critically injured patients were massively edematous, being ventilated with 1 liter tidal volumes and frequently required prone positioning. Multiple organ failure was common, and its etiology in trauma was a long way from being clearly understood.

Trauma resuscitation, critical care support, and early survival had advanced enough by the 1970s that MOF occurred in relatively large numbers of trauma-tized patients. Early epidemiologic studies highlighted the association of infection and systemic sepsis with MOF and a causal relationship in the development of MOF was inferred. For much of the 1970s and 1980s, research focused on occult infection, bacterial translocation, and postinjury immunosuppression as engines driving MOF.[8-10] At that time, very limited literature established any relationship between the severity of injury and tissue perfusion to the subse-quent development of MOF.[11] In part, due to the size of their study (394 patients was very large for the time), they established the importance of tissue injury and hypoperfusion in MOF, predicting its development from parameters present at admission or within 12–24 hours.

The overall mortality for the 529 patients admitted to Denver General Hospital greater than 16 years old with ISS > 15 was 33%, high compared to today's outcomes. Today, mortality for patients with the same criteria at Vanderbilt University Medical Center is half that (15.8%). So, what has changed since 1994? The ARDS Network published their landmark study on low tidal volume ventilation in 2000,[12] and since then, advancement of trauma systems, balanced resuscitation and limitation of crystalloids, glycemic control, antibiotic-coated catheters, and early nutrition, to name a few. This seminal work provided critical building blocks for our subsequent advancements in the resuscitation of critically injured patients.

REFERENCES

1. Sauaia A, Moore FA, Moore EE, Haenel JB, Read RA, Lezotte DC. Early predictors of postinjury multiple organ failure. *Arch Surg.* 1994; 129(1): 39–45.
2. American College of Surgeons Committee on Trauma Blue Book. 2007.
3. Feliciano DV. 50 years of trauma, burns, and surgical critical care at the Southwestern Surgical Congress. *Am J Surg.* 1998; 175(3A Suppl): 99S–107S.
4. Aggarwal BB, Gupta SC, Kim JH. Historical perspectives on tumor necrosis factor and its superfamily: 25 years later, a golden journey. *Blood.* 2012; 119(3): 651–665.
5. Kishimoto T. Interleukin-6: Discovery of a pleiotropic cytokine. *Arthritis Res Ther.* 2006; 8(Suppl 2): S2.
6. Eddy VA, Key SP, Morris JA, Jr. Abdominal compartment syndrome: Etiology, detection, and management. *J Tenn Med Assoc.* 1994; 87(2): 55–57.
7. Rotondo MF, Schwab CW, McGonigal MD, et al. 'Damage control': An approach for improved survival in exsanguinating penetrating abdominal injury. *J Trauma.* 1993; 35(3): 375–382.

8. Moore FA, Moore EE. Evolving concepts in the pathogenesis of postinjury multiple organ failure. *Surg Clin North Am.* 1995; 75(2): 257–277.
9. Saadia R. Trauma and bacterial translocation. *Br J Surg.* 1995; 82(9): 1243–1244.
10. Sauaia A, Moore FA, Moore EE, Haenel JB, Read RA. Pneumonia: Cause or symptom of postinjury multiple organ failure? *Am J Surg.* 1993; 166(6): 606–610.
11. Roumen RM, Redl H, Schlag G, Sandtner W, Koller W, Goris RJ. Scoring systems and blood lactate concentrations in relation to the development of adult respiratory distress syndrome and multiple organ failure in severely traumatized patients. *J Trauma.* 1993; 35(3): 349–355.
12. Brower RG, Matthay MA, Morris A, Schoenfeld D, Thompson BT, Wheeler A. Ventilation with lower tidal volumes as compared with traditional tidal volumes for acute lung injury and the acute respiratory distress syndrome. *N Engl J Med.* 2000; 342(18): 1301–1308.

Editor Notes: This paper retrospectively reviewed the outcomes of patients ISS > 15 who survived more than 24 hours. Risk factors for multiple organ failure were identified: age over 55, ISS over 24, more than 6 units packed red cells. In addition, development of a metabolic acidosis manifest as a persistent base deficit or lactic acidosis was associated with organ failure. This was one of the first studies to help identify predictors of organ dysfunction after trauma, some of which could be impacted upon the clinician (base deficit, lactate, transfusion volume).

Limitations:

Retrospective analysis;
Single center experience;
Limited population size;
Cohort study;
Definition of multiple organ failure was different from what clinicians typically use today.

CHAPTER 47

Alcohol Interventions in a Trauma Center as a Means of Reducing the Risk of Injury Recurrence

Gentilello LM, Rivara FP, Donovan DM, Jurkovich GJ,
Daranciang E, Dunn CW, Villaveces A, Copass M, Ries RR.

Ann Surg 230(4):473–480; discussion 480–483, 1999

Abstract   This paper attempts to address an increasing worldwide trend in alcohol consumption in all ages and its huge impact on trauma-related death, injury, disability, and national and international health-related expenditure.

Objective   Alcoholism is the leading risk factor for injury. The authors hypothesized that providing brief alcohol interventions as a routine component of trauma care would significantly reduce alcohol consumption and would decrease the rate of trauma recidivism.

Methods   This study was a randomized, prospective controlled trial in a level I trauma center. Patients were screened using a blood alcohol concentration, gamma glutamyl transpeptidase level, and Short Michigan Alcoholism Screening Test (SMAST). Those with positive results were randomized to a brief intervention or control group. Reinjury was detected by a computerized search of emergency department and statewide hospital discharge records, and 6- and 12-month interviews were conducted to assess alcohol use.

Results   A total of 2,524 patients were screened; 1,153 screened positive (46%). Three hundred sixty-six were randomized to the intervention group, and 396 to controls. At 12 months, the intervention group decreased alcohol consumption by 21.8 ± 3.7 drinks per week; in the control group, the decrease was 6.7 ± 5.8 (p = 0.03). The reduction was most apparent in patients with mild to moderate alcohol problems (SMAST score 3–8); they had 21.6 ± 4.2 fewer drinks per week, compared to an increase of 2.3 ± 8.3 drinks per week in controls (p < 0.01). There was a 47% reduction in injuries requiring either emergency department or trauma center admission (hazard ratio 0.53, 95% confidence interval 0.26 to 1.07, p = 0.07) and a 48% reduction in injuries requiring hospital admission (3 years follow-up).

Conclusions   Alcohol interventions are associated with a reduction in alcohol intake and a reduced risk of trauma recidivism. Given the prevalence of alcohol problems in trauma centers, screening, intervention, and counseling for alcohol problems should be routine.

Author Commentary by Larry M. Gentilello

The 1966 publication of the historic paper, "Accidental Injury: The Neglected Disease of Modern Society," is cited as the inaugural step in the development of trauma centers in the United States. Within a decade, the American College of Surgeons followed with the publication of the first edition of *Optimal Hospital Resources for Care of the Seriously Injured Patient*, which summarized the essential characteristics of a trauma system. Without a doubt, the establishment of trauma systems was one of the most important developments not just in surgery, but also in the history of medicine.

Subsequent research, where injury mortality was compared in two similar counties, proved the importance of trauma systems. All patients in San Francisco County were brought to a trauma center, while in Orange County patients were transported to the nearest hospital. Overall, 41% of the patients taken to the nearest hospital died from a preventable or possibly preventable cause, while only one death in San Francisco County was so judged (1.1%).

While challenges in the distribution of trauma centers remain, mainly in rural areas, by 2010 over 90% of the population in the United States had access to a trauma center within 60 minutes "Golden Hour." When the rate of death associated with any disease decreases by such a dramatic amount (41%–1%), it is not an overstatement to describe it as one of the most important developments in the history of health care.

Since the development of the first trauma center, it has always been known that the leading cause of injuries has been alcohol misuse. When drugs are also considered, the majority of patients who present to a trauma center are found to be under the influence of a substance that impaired their reaction time, safety, and judgment.

Until 10 years ago, trauma centers always treated the injury and ignored the underlying cause. The risk of injury recurrence, trauma center readmission, or subsequent injury-related death was high. When a patient suffering from a myocardial infarction is admitted to a coronary care unit, physicians always investigate whether or not there is underlying hypertension, hyperlipidemia, or some other treatable risk factor. All patients admitted to a pulmonary care unit are screened for tobacco use. It was time for trauma centers to take a similar approach.

Most patients who sustain an alcohol-related injury are not addicted or dependent on alcohol. They were intoxicated, usually as a result of a binge, overuse, or simply not being aware of the risks they were taking. The principle underlying this paper was that words such as, "alcoholism" and "alcohol abuse"—words still heard on hospital wards—do not apply to most trauma patients. These words are not even in the current *DSM-V*.

Similar to most medical conditions, such as hypertension, diabetes, or COPD, there is a spectrum, with patients sometimes having no symptoms, or having mild, moderate, or severe symptoms. The majority of patients admitted to a trauma center do not have severe symptoms and benefit from skillfully provided advice about how to better manage the risks and rewards of using substances that affect their injury risk.

In this prospective, controlled, randomized study, a 15-minute intervention, and subsequent follow-up letter, led to a nearly 50% reduction in injury-related emergency department visits and hospital admissions, with up to 5 years of follow-up. In 2006, the American College of Surgeons Committee on Trauma (COT) adopted alcohol screening and intervention as criteria for trauma center verification.

The following year the Centers for Disease Control awarded the COT the Injury Control and Health Impact Award in recognition that this was the first time in the history of medicine that any mandate or requirement had ever been passed requiring physicians to address substance misuse or any other problem that might be related to mental health.

Expert Commentary by Asaf A. Gave

Over the years, we made little progress in reducing the incidence of alcohol-related injuries and had no influence on preventive interventions. A brief, cheap, and efficient intervention as demonstrated in this article may reduce recurrent trauma by approximately 50%.

The recent reorganization of the trauma system in the United States presents an opportunity for a national initiative in all level I and level II trauma centers for a "brief intervention" to reduce alcohol-related morbidity and mortality. This idea may also be expanded to the younger population as well.

In many states obtaining BAC (blood alcohol concentration) from vehicular trauma patients is routine, and devising an alcohol consumption screening tool is easy to adapt and simple to administer. Having a "brief intervention"-trained consultant as a member of the trauma team may reduce the number of trauma-related hospital beds by half and national trauma admissions by 1.8 million. Also reducing alcohol-related mortality in drunk drivers and drunk pedestrians from 40%–20%.

This paper clearly demonstrated that with simple intervention we can make a great impact in preventing future alcohol-related trauma, especially in mild and moderate alcohol users.

Editor Notes: The authors used a randomized controlled trial to demonstrate in this unique landmark study that a short (30-minute) simple counseling intervention following a positive alcohol screening test, could be beneficial in reducing alcohol intake and the likelihood of subsequent trauma admissions. In 752 trauma patients, those receiving the brief intervention had a dramatic decrease in weekly drinks and a nearly 50% diminution in the frequency of injuries requiring hospital admission over the following 3 years.

Limitations:

Primarily young male population;
Baseline data not obtained on 55% of control group;
The intervention group could have received more care than simple intervention as not a blinded study (for example, the follow-up letter one month after discharge could have had an impact);
Self-reported alcohol consumption information may be faulty;
Unclear as to why the intervention resulted in decreased risk-taking behavior in general;
Lack of benefit in chronic alcohol drinkers.

CHAPTER 48

Post-Traumatic Stress Disorder in Vietnam Veterans

Kolb LC. N Engl J Med 314(10):641–642, 1986

Abstract In Kolb's seminal 1986 *New England Journal of Medicine* paper,[1] he noted the many comorbidities of PTSD including insomnia, chronic pain, substance use disorders, and suicide. In a previous publication, Kolb had been one of the first to report that combat trauma can result in abnormal conditioned emotional and physiological responses.[2] These reactions can include episodic increases in heart rate, blood pressure, and muscle tension that can lead to long-term increases in morbidity and mortality. He also highlighted abnormalities in catecholamine and cortisol excretion reactions that may denote a permanent impairment of central neuronal functioning.[3]

Expert Commentary Alan L. Peterson

Some of the greatest discoveries in medicine and science have come from the military battlefield. Deployed military trauma surgeons have made many of these innovations and advancements. Although there has been less of an emphasis on the psychiatric sequelae of combat trauma, a landmark manuscript by the visionary psychiatrist Lawrence Kolb[1] highlighted the excessive psychosocial distress and increased mortality of men who served in combat during the Vietnam War. Many of Kolb's initial insights regarding combat-related post-traumatic stress disorder (PTSD) came from his experiences in the assessment and treatment of patients with "battle fatigue" as a US Navy psychiatrist during World War II. This helped spur a career in academic medicine with an emphasis in combat-related PTSD. Kolb was also one of the pioneers to investigate phantom limb pain after traumatic amputations.[4–6]

Kolb's landmark paper also described how the American societal denigration of Vietnam veterans led them to social isolation and resentment of health care providers and institutions—especially the Veterans Health Administration (VHA). Early opportunities for detection, referral, and treatment of PTSD were lost and likely exacerbated the long-term psychological and physical health impact of exposure to combat-related trauma. Kolb helped stimulate decades of research on the assessment and treatment of combat-related PTSD and prompted improvements in policy and practice. Three years after his landmark manuscript, the National Center for PTSD was established by the Department of Veterans Affairs in 1989 to address the needs of veterans and other trauma survivors with PTSD.

Fast-forward 30 years and we face similar challenges in a new generation of combat veterans who have deployed since November 9, 2001, in support of the Global War on Terrorism. Only recently have the first randomized clinical trials been completed on the treatment of combat-related PTSD in active duty military personnel. Most of these studies were conducted by the Department of Defense-funded STRONG STAR Consortium (South Texas Research Organizational Network Guiding Studies on Trauma and Resilience). STRONG STAR, headquartered in San Antonio, Texas, includes the collaboration of over 100 nationwide investigators and over 30 military, civilian, and VHA institutions. These studies have demonstrated that combat-related PTSD can be effectively treated with non-pharmacological cognitive behavioral therapies, such as cognitive processing therapy,[7,8] prolonged exposure therapy,[9] and abbreviated treatments using behavioral health consultants integrated into primary care settings.[10–12] However, similar to Kolb's conclusion over three decades ago, much more research is still needed on the causes, prevention, and treatment of PTSD.

REFERENCES

1. Kolb LC. Post-traumatic stress disorder in Vietnam veterans. *N Engl J Med*. 1986; 314(10): 641–642.
2. Kolb LC. The post-traumatic stress disorders of combat: A subgroup with a conditioned emotional response. *Mil Med*. 1984; 149(5): 237–243.
3. Pallmeyer TP, Blanchard EB, Kolb LC. The psychophysiology of combat-induced post-traumatic stress disorder in Vietnam veterans. *Behav Res Ther*. 1986; 24(6): 645–652.
4. Kolb LC. Psychiatric aspects of treatment for intractable pain in the phantom limb. *Med Clin North Am*. 1950; 34(4): 1029–1041.
5. Kolb LC. Psychiatric aspects of treatment of the painful phantom limb. *Proc Staff Meet Mayo Clin*. 1950; 25(16): 467–471.
6. Kolb LC, Frank LM, Watson EJ. Treatment of the acute painful phantom limb. *Proc Staff Meet Mayo Clin*. 1952; 27(6): 110–118.
7. Resick PA, Wachen JS, Mintz J, et al. A randomized clinical trial of group cognitive processing therapy compared with group present-centered therapy for PTSD among active duty military personnel. *J Consult Clin Psychol*. 2015; 83(6): 1058–1068. doi:10.1037/ccp0000016.
8. Resick PA, Wachen JS, Dondanville KA, et al. Effect of group vs individual cognitive processing therapy in active-duty military seeking treatment for posttraumatic stress disorder: A randomized clinical trial. *JAMA Psych*. 2017; 74(1): 28–36. doi:10.1001/jamapsychiatry.2016.2729.
9. Foa EB, McLean CP, Zang Y, et al. Effect of prolonged exposure cognitive behavioral therapy delivered over 2 weeks vs 8 weeks vs present centered therapy on PTSD severity in military personnel: A randomized clinical trial. Under Review.
10. Cigrang JA, Rauch SA, Avila LL, Bryan CJ, Goodie JL, Hryshko-Mullen A, Peterson AL, & the STRONG STAR Consortium. Treatment of active-duty military with PTSD in primary care: Early findings. *Psych Services*. 2011; 8(2): 104–113. doi:10.1037/a0022740

11. Cigrang JA, Rauch SA, Mintz J, Brundige A, Avila LL, Bryan CJ, Goodie JL, Peterson AL; STRONG STAR Consortium. Treatment of active duty military with PTSD in primary care: A follow-up report. *J Anxiety Disord.* 2015; 36: 110–114. doi:10.1016/j.janxdis.2015.10.003.

12. Cigrang JA, Rauch SA, Mintz J, et al. Moving effective treatment for posttraumatic stress disorder to primary care: A randomized controlled trial with active duty military. *Fam Syst Health.* 2017; 35(4): 450–462. doi:10.1037/fsh0000315.

Expert Commentary by Alexander L. Eastman

The trauma and critical care surgeon often stands between life and death. As well as the stress associated with the clinical care of patients in crisis, providers in these arenas also encounter the added stress associated with complicated family dynamics, difficult social circumstances and other professional and personal obligations that may be at play. Making matters worse, stress of all types is associated with profound degradation in human performance. Providers in these specialties do not like to appear weak or susceptible to things that others might succumb to and hence the perfect storm is present. As such, we should take it as fact that there is untreated PTSD present in the house of trauma and critical care. In this landmark article by Kolb,[1] his characterization of the scourge of PTSD in Vietnam combat veterans, as well as its indolent course made worse by unwarranted stigma, could as easily describe some of our nation's trauma surgeons, emergency physicians, and first responders. It is likely that some of our colleagues are suffering and performing at far less than optimal—both of which should be correctible with recognition and simple intervention. In short, we must do a much better job of caring for each other.

Caring for other human beings is challenging, yet caring for them in times of crisis can be brutal. Defined as the emotions and behaviors that a person experiences as the result of being exposed to another's traumatic experience, secondary traumatic stress (STS) should be part of the essential job description of nearly everyone in our business.

Consider the core symptoms and take a minute of honest reflection—how many of us can say that during our careers we have *never* felt one of them? Far more of us have experienced these symptoms than ever admit to it.

While a number of reports and surveys have attempted to quantify the presence of PTSD in the trauma community, there is a certain stigma attached with the use of the word *disorder*. Joseph et al. surveyed members of both the American Association for the Surgery of Trauma (AAST) and the Eastern Association for the Surgery of Trauma (EAST)—both national trauma organizations.[2] More than 40% (*n* = 181) showed symptoms of PTSD, and 15%

($n = 68$) met the *DSM-V* criteria for PTSD. Male surgeons, operating more than 15 cases per month, having more than seven call duties per month, and having less than 4 hours of relaxation per day all were at risk for the development of PTSD.

PTSD in trauma surgeons is a potential sleeping epidemic among us that likely has long-standing effects on our friends and colleagues that in most programs and institutions is simply ignored at best or minimized/stigmatized at worst. The deleterious effects of the work that we do likely persists in trauma surgeons, emergency physicians, nurses, and across the spectrum of disaster responders. In order to become truly resilient organizations and providers, we must recognize this to be a problem, must have frank and honest discourse, and must adapt programs that have proven to be effective. Only when we have accomplished each of these goals will our critical personnel and programs be truly at their most effective place.

REFERENCES

1. Kolb LC. Post-traumatic stress disorder in Vietnam veterans. *N Engl J Med*. 1986; 314(10): 641–642.
2. Joseph B, Pandit V, Hadeed G, et al. Unveiling posttraumatic stress disorder in trauma surgeons: A national survey. *J Trauma Acute Care Surg*. 2014; 77: 148–154.

Editor Notes: This was one of the first applications of this relatively new term "post-traumatic stress disorder" or PTSD to combat veterans. Mental illness had long been recognized following war experiences, but this essay was felt to be a seminal paper in the field. There was no data reported, just a description of the entity and why it is felt to be important.

Limitations:

No data, no validation, observational experience reported in narrative form.

CHAPTER 49

Outcome after Major Trauma: 12-Month and 18-Month Follow-Up Results from the Trauma Recovery Project

Holbrook TL, Anderson JP, Sieber WJ, Browner D, Hoyt DB.

J Trauma 46(5):765–771; discussion 771–773, 1999

Abstract   This manuscript is an early attempt to study post-discharge outcomes of trauma patients, a subject that even now receives inadequate attention and emphasis. This qualifies as a landmark publication for many reasons. These include the obvious (and as it turns out, prescient) value of a report on post-discharge outcomes, especially at a time our profession was (appropriately) focused on prehospital and inpatient care challenges of delivering patients quickly to the right facility and saving their lives. Without reliable data on longer-term outcomes, however, it would be difficult to determine the true value of the frequently complex and expensive care we provide. The authors use of a validated measure of wellness, the incorporation of non-physical injury into outcome assessment, and the inclusion of an entire cohort of patients are also noteworthy. Although the modern-day concept of "patient-centered care" was not commonly discussed at that time, this work draws attention to the importance of patients' assessment of their well-being and the quality of their life postinjury.

Background   The importance of outcome after major injury has continued to gain attention in light of the ongoing development of sophisticated trauma care systems in the United States. The Trauma Recovery Project (TRP) is a large prospective epidemiologic study designed to examine multiple outcomes after major trauma in adults aged 18 years and older, including quality of life, functional outcome, and psychologic sequelae, such as depression and post-traumatic stress disorder (PTSD). Patient outcomes were assessed at discharge and at 6, 12, and 18 months after discharge. The specific objectives of the present report are to describe functional outcomes at the 12-month and 18-month follow-ups in the TRP population and to examine the association of putative risk factors with functional outcome.

Methods   Between December 1, 1993 and September 1, 1996, 1,048 eligible trauma patients triaged to four participating trauma center hospitals in the San Diego Regionalized Trauma System were enrolled in the TRP study. The admission criteria for patients were as follows: (1) age 18 years or older; (2) Glasgow Coma Scale score on admission of 12 or greater; and (3) length of stay greater than 24 hours. Functional outcome after trauma was measured before and after injury using the Quality of Well-Being (QWB) Scale, an index sensitive to the well end of the functioning continuum (0 = death, 1.000 = optimum functioning). Follow-up at 12 months after discharge was completed for 806 patients (79%), and follow-up at 18 months was completed for 780 patients (74%). Follow-up contact at any of the study time points (6, 12, or 18 months) was achieved for 926 (88%) patients.

Results   The mean age was 36 ± 14.8 years, and 70% of the patients were male; 52% were white, 30% were Hispanic, and 18% were black or other. Less than 40% of study participants were married or living together. The mean Injury Severity Score was 13 ± 8.5, with 85% blunt injuries and a mean length of stay of 7 ± 9.2 days. QWB scores before injury reflected the norm for a healthy adult population (mean, 0.810 ± 0.171). At the 12-month follow-up, there were very high levels of functional limitation (QWB mean score, 0.670 ± 0.137). Only 18% of patients followed at 12 months had scores above 0.800, the norm for a healthy population. There was no improvement in functional limitation at the 18-month follow-up (QWB mean score, 0.678 ± 0.130). The majority of patients (80%) at the 18-month follow-up continued to have QWB scores below the healthy norm of 0.800. Postinjury depression, PTSD, serious extremity injury, and intensive care unit days were significant independent predictors of 12-month and 18-month QWB outcome.

Conclusions   This study demonstrates a prolonged and profound level of functional limitation after major trauma at 12-month and 18-month follow-up. This is the first report of long-term outcome based on the QWB Scale, a standardized quality-of-life measure, and provides new and provocative evidence that the magnitude of dysfunction after major injury has been underestimated. Postinjury depression, PTSD, serious extremity injury, and intensive care unit days are significantly associated with 12-month and 18-month QWB outcomes.

Expert Commentary by Ronald Simon

Presented at the 58th Annual Meeting of the American Association for the Surgery of Trauma, this paper was one of the most remarkable papers presented that year. You can always tell by the comments following the presentation whether a paper was scientifically valid or impactful. In the case of this paper, the comments all noted the quality and value of the paper. Almost 3 years before the groundbreaking *New England Journal of Medicine* article by Bosse and MacKenzie[1] on the effects of severe lower extremity injury on functional outcomes, this study scientifically reviewed the impact of injury on overall well-being. It not only represented an example of high-quality research, it finally confirmed what many of us believed, but had never been confirmed with as rigorous a protocol and data set as presented here. While we all knew the statistics on morbidity, mortality, and the immediate toll of being injured, this paper confirmed, in the most rigorous fashion to date, that saving someone's life does not mean that their life will return to their preinjury status.

This prospective, multi-institutional study was the highest quality of evidence of the long-term consequences of injury on well-being. With 1,000 patients enrolled and a 74% follow-up rate at 18 months, this study was unusually powerful. The authors achieved this ambitious goal by creating the Trauma Recovery Project, which collected data from four trauma centers in San Diego County.

It was obvious that patients with severe brain and spine injuries would never return to their previous lives, but what about people with less devastating injuries? This paper demonstrated that life does not return to its previous state in many people with more moderate injuries (average ISS was 13 ± 8.5) and, by only including patients with GCS > 12 on admission, it eliminated patients with severe brain injury. Using the Quality of Well-Being (QWB) index, this paper showed the long-term physical and social effects of being injured. The QWB is a composite index of three major indicators: mobility, physical activity, and social activity. The QWB, at the time, was the best method for evaluating the desired outcomes. The authors showed that at 6, 12, and 18 months post injury over 40% of those studied never returned to preinjury levels of well-being. Interestingly and counterintuitively, there was little improvement in scores after 6 months.

Risk factors for the decrease in well-being included: Postinjury depression, PTSD, extremity injury with AIS ≥ 3, and ICU length of stay (LOS). Although others had shown that the lack of a social support structure decreased well-being post injury, this study did not support that finding.

REFERENCE

1. Bosse MJ, MacKenzie EJ, Kellam JF, et al. An analysis of outcomes of reconstruction or amputation of leg-threatening injuries. *N Engl J Med*. 2002; 347: 1924–1931.

Expert Commentary by Samir M. Fakhry

Returning patients to their preinjury status turns out to be much harder than getting them discharged alive from the hospital, the short-term goal most clinicians seek. In fact, this research pointed out that nearly half (42%) of the patients had not returned to their preinjury status at 18 months follow-up. This has been substantiated by others and may not represent totally unexpected news to experienced trauma professionals, then or now. What was unexpected was that the strongest correlates to poor outcome were depression and PTSD at discharge or 6 months and not the markers of severity of physical injury. The only physical finding that approached depression and PTSD in significance was extremity injury.

That non-physical dysfunction was so highly correlated with worse outcomes strikes me as the seminal contribution of this research.

A significant body of work now confirms that many trauma patients report emotional or psychological distress after injury (19%−42%) and that this is associated with deficits in physical recovery, social functioning, and quality of life. Because follow-up care after injury is limited, many acute care providers do not realize that so many injured patients do poorly after hospital discharge and that non-physical injury appears to be a major contributor to poor outcomes.

The corollary is that better follow-up care, especially for depression, PTSD, and other non-physical injury, has the potential to improve quality of life and save billions of dollars annually in lost productivity. Research has already provided the majority of knowledge needed to achieve this goal. A growing awareness of this need is evident in the 2014 publication of the *Resources for Optimal Care of the Injured Patient*, the first of six editions to recommend consideration of center-based screening and referral for treatment of PTSD and depression. However, relatively few US trauma centers monitor and address non-physical recovery. As a result, up to 90% of patients who stand to benefit from mental health treatment after traumatic injury do not receive it. This call to action from almost 20 years ago still awaits.

Editor Notes: This is one of the few long-term outcome studies of trauma patients. This prospective investigation demonstrated a persistence of diminution of quality of life following trauma. This alteration was profound and related to the severity of injury.

Limitations:

Relatively short follow-up time period (18 months);
Limited baseline quality of life data for comparison (i.e: preinjury status unclear);
Relatively small population;
Patients were mostly young (mean age 36).

CHAPTER 50

Battle Injuries of the Arteries in World War II: An Analysis of 2,471 Cases

DeBakey ME, Simeone FA. Ann Surg 123(4):534–579, 1946

Abstract   This seminal work represents a major undertaking on the part of DeBakey and Simeone and its impact has been profound on the progression of battlefield and civilian vascular trauma management. Their work stems from recognition that in the combat setting, no satisfactory methods for managing arterial injuries existed and there was a lack of unanimity regarding management of these injuries or choice of techniques for individual injuries. They realized that this was compounded by a lack of outcome data for these injuries in previous conflicts. In their analysis, the authors made comparisons to significant data collected in previous wars.

Expert Commentary by Brian J. Eastridge

The management of war wounds has driven advancements in medicine since the beginning of recorded history. In fact, Hippocrates proposed "… he who would be a surgeon should follow the army …" During the American Civil War, the primary therapy for extremity vascular injury was amputation. Surgeons were generally loathed and referred to as "butchers of the battlefield." World War I ushered in an era of improved evacuation, resuscitation, and anesthesia. Major vascular injuries were frequently managed by ligation or wound closure; however, these wounds were associated with a high rate of soft tissue infection and the ultimate outcomes of combat vascular injury remained largely unchanged as most of these ligations ended in death or amputation. Similar to previous wars, World War II manifested advantages to combat casualties including antisepsis, antibiosis, and resuscitation with blood and plasma. Additionally, partly at the urging of COL Michael DeBakey, Special Surgical Consultant to the Surgeon General of the Army, the US military developed a fundamental understanding of the value of medical data, which formed the early roots of evidence-based combat casualty care.

DeBakey and Simeone described a series of 2,471 vascular injuries sustained in battle during World War II. They saw that the majority of the vessel injuries managed surgically at theater hospitals were brachial, femoral, popliteal, and tibial in origin. Vascular injuries were managed almost exclusively with ligation that was associated with an amputation rate of 49%. Simple arterial repair with lateral arteriorrhaphy or end to end anastomosis was attempted in 81 casualties with a substantially lower amputation rate of 36%. The presentation of the data was a relatively simple analysis, and, in fact, the final conclusion was unenthusiastic about the approach of acute repair for the management of vascular injury on the battlefield. However, the study and its extended implications have had a profound impact on the advancement of injury care.

The study fostered the advancement of vascular surgery as a specialty discipline of surgery as well as a lineage of military vascular surgeons, including Dr. Carl Hughes (Korea), Dr. Norman Rich (Vietnam), Dr. Todd Rasmussen (Enduring Freedom/Iraqi Freedom), and others who have carried the torch and driven significant advances and innovation in trauma vascular surgery. Postulating that the anatomic morphology of injuries was isolated to small- to medium-sized arteries was driven by the fact that casualties with larger vessel injuries likely did not survive evacuation due to poorly positioned surgical assets. This 70-year-old insight was a premonition of current efforts to develop a military trauma system and a comprehensive understanding of the implications of prehospital mortality on the battlefield. Likewise, the perception that arterial repair was associated with improved outcomes was tempered by the observations that the procedure required advanced technical skill, which most surgeons did not possess. Additionally, combat casualty care survival was often predicated upon often delayed evacuation in the context of destructive polytrauma and extensive blood loss that took precedence over definitive vascular repair ... a concept we recognize today as Damage Control.

Expert Commentary by John Kennedy Bini

DeBakey and Simeone systematically collected data on 2,471 acute arterial injuries occurring during wwii. They focused on incidence, types, location, morbidity, methods of management, and factors influencing outcomes. The authors also addressed the limitations of performing vascular surgery in the austere environment and the impact that delays in casualty evacuation had on limb salvage. Recognition of these logistic limitations has significantly impacted improvements in casualty evacuation and the distribution of surgical resources in order to reduce the time from injury to surgical care.

DeBakey and Simeone looked extensively at the wound characteristics and how they impacted outcomes, in particular amputation rates. They recognized and published that destructive soft tissue injuries, fractures, location of the injury, and concomitant venous injury significantly and negatively impacted outcomes and should be taken into consideration prior to heroic attempts at arterial salvage. Despite over 70 years of advancement in technology, these issues still impact vascular trauma decision making in both the military and civilian settings.

DeBakey and Simeone recognized that hemorrhage control and management of shock were priorities and took precedence over arterial repair and limb salvage. They also realized that limb outcomes were dependent upon temporizing distal perfusion. This is the foundation of modern damage control vascular surgery and the use of temporary vascular shunts. In doing so, the authors challenged existing dogma regarding the performance of sympathectomy and routine ligation of uninjured paired major veins.

The most significant impact of this work was the authors' recognition that improvements in care could only take place with robust data collection and analysis. With this recognition, they established the first formal vascular injury registry and in doing so, established a heritage of military vascular surgeons who built upon their work, collected data, and improved the care of trauma patients in the combat and civilian environments. Carl Hughes captured Korean War vascular injury data as we progressed from routine ligation to vascular repair. Norman Rich created the Vietnam Vascular Registry. These lessons learned were carried forward to the recent conflicts in Iraq and Afghanistan. Todd Rasmussen's development of the Balad Vascular Registry in Iraq led to the Global War on Terror Vascular Initiative and contributed significantly to the establishment of the Joint Theatre Trauma Registry, which is now the DoD Trauma Registry. In an attempt to bring these lessons learned to civilian vascular trauma, Joe Dubose and Todd Rasmussen have partnered with the AAST to establish the PROspective Observational Vascular Injury Treatment (PROOVIT) database to prospectively collect robust data on civilian vascular trauma. With this current living initiative, the work of DeBakey and Simeone is not only landmark, but to date, immortal.

Editor Notes: The authors describe the military medical experience during World War II with nearly 2,500 arterial injuries and compare these results with previous conflicts. They found a higher amputation rate was associated with more distal injuries (popliteal), combination of arterial plus venous injuries, long delays to reperfusion (> than 10 hours), and described the value of extremity compartment fasciotomy. This represents one of the first uses of a huge trauma database to understand the management of a focused topic (in this case vascular injury during wartime) and delineate potential opportunities for improvement in the future.

Limitations:

Potential for underreporting of the most and least severe injuries;
Paper database;
Certainty that many combat wounded did not survive to medical care and accurate diagnosis because of very long transport times, limited medical availability, and potential for missed injuries in those without autopsy.

Index

A

Abbreviated Injury Scale (AIS), 11–12
abdominal cavity, 114, 123, 171
abdominal compartment syndrome
    (ACS), 114
  diagnosis and management, 184
  fascial prosthesis, 182
  IAP, 183
  MOF, 204–205
  OAM, 182–183
  signs, 181
abdominal GSWs
  kinetic energy, 173–174
  management, 171
  mandatory operation policy, 173
  manuscript, 172
  penetrating wounds, 173–174
  principles of care, 173
  safety and cost-effectiveness, 172
  SNOM, 172
  statements, 171
abdominal trauma
  anesthesia, 81
  CT scans, 85–87
  description, 82
  gunshot wounds, 82–83
  hemodynamic instability, 82
  KCHC, 81
  management, 82–83
  patient observation, 83
  stab wounds, 81–82
acetabular fractures, 175–176, 179
acidosis
  blood pressure, 21
  gut mucosal, 181–182
  hemorrhagic shock, 19
  hypotension, 22
  IAP measurements, 181
ACS, *see* abdominal compartment
  syndrome

adult respiratory distress syndrome
  (ARDS), 142–143, 175, 178
Advanced Trauma Life Support (ATLS®)
  course, 43–44
Advanced Trauma Operative Management
  (ATOM) course, 125
Agarwal, Suresh "Mitu, 64–65
Air Force Theater Hospital
  (AFTH), 146
Alam, HB, 45–47
alcohol interventions in trauma center
  abuse, 211
  alcoholism, 209, 211
  BAC, 209, 211
  development, 210
  intake, 210
  SMAST, 209
American Association for the Surgery
  of Trauma (AAST), 82, 86, 129, 182,
  215, 223
anaerobes, 195
anesthesia, 81, 125, 187
angioembolization, 167–168
angiographic embolization (AE),
  133–134, 163
Annals of Surgery (journal),
  115, 166
antero-posterior compression (APC),
  175–178
anti-anaerobic agents, 195
antibiotics
  PAT, 195–197
  prophylactic, 193–194
  SSI, 193
antifibrinolytics, 32
aortic endografts, 151
API, *see* arterial pressure index
Archives of Surgery (journal), 172
arterial bleeding, 114, 137–138
arterial injuries, 221–223

Printed in the United States
by Baker & Taylor Publisher Services

Printed in the United States
by Baker & Taylor Publisher Services